A Pound of Prevention: Eight Secrets of Healthy Living

Dr. Alfred Nkut

AuthorHouse™
1663 Liberty Drive
Bloomington, IN 47403
www.authorhouse.com
Phone: 1-800-839-8640

First published by AuthorHouse   2/4/2011

ISBN: 978-1-4567-4129-7 (sc)
ISBN: 978-1-4567-4127-3 (e)

Library of Congress Control Number: 2011905921

Dedicated to my parents, Susan Amembo and Joseph Ndenkeh.

Acknowledgments

Thank you to Lisa Lepage for proof reading my manual and making very insightful suggestions!

Contents

Foreword

My experience as a primary care doctor has taught me that the eight elements presented in this book are the essence of how we can improve the status of our health. I call them *secrets* because I am now revealing them to you: your secrets for success healthy living.

Quite a few observations prompted me to write this book. The fact is that health care facilities, including clinics and emergency rooms, are overcrowded with people suffering from minor ailments. I have come to learn that for such people, the dilemma is that they do not know how serious their symptoms are. I thought that I could drastically reduce overcrowding, and also save peoples' valuable time, if they learned how to use the "downhill rule," a technique that I use to assess the severity of peoples' medical problems. (You'll find the explanation of this rule in Chapter Four.)

Quite a few people have benefited from using this rule to successfully assess chest pain and viral illnesses to see whether an expert opinion is needed. Now I'm making this information available to more people in this book.

I find that many patients are knowledgeable about what to do in order to improve their health status. For example, they understand the benefits of regular exercise and eating properly. The problem is that they lack the motivation and discipline to act. That is why this book is more motivational than instructional. It will help you reduce the gap between knowledge and action, with the net result of improving your health status.

You will learn how to develop a disciplined lifestyle in order to bridge the gap between knowledge and action. Using weight management as an example, you will have to resist the urge to overindulge with willpower. Why? Because willpower is the basis of discipline.

I have also observed that men are more neglectful of taking care of their health than women. Men are more likely to take their car to the garage for regular checkups than to go and see their doctor! Is that not amazing? I believe that if people understand why such checkups are necessary, they may be more inclined to go for them. Even if you are diagnosed with a disease, you're better off identifying it early, because then you stand a better chance of recovering or surviving the disease. And remember, the frequency of regular checkups will depend on a number of things, including age and medical status, which is discussed in more detail in Chapter Five.

Health promotion still remains the best option to foster good health, especially given the fact that some health problems could lead to permanent damage. For example, a stroke may leave someone paralyzed for life. And strokes can potentially be prevented by learning how to control stress levels or by simply stopping at a health clinic to get blood pressure checked. There is no question that it is easier to maintain good health than to try to regain it!

Most of what is involved in staying healthy is doing the basic things that are common knowledge to most people. But you make the difference by not only knowing what to do but putting into practice.

Good health is not just the absence of disease. It is a spectrum that reflects one's level of functioning and happiness. Why? Because in general, we can do whatever we want and call that success. But it must lead to personal fulfillment, which I think is the great prize of good health.

Therefore, for optimum health, there has to be balance and harmony between mind, body, and spirit. The spirit is the immortal part of a human being, our internal and natural source of happiness. Much of our happiness is determined by the quality of our thoughts. So learning how to arrange your mind and detoxify it from toxic or negative emotions is also an important part of staying healthy.

The purpose of this book is to show you how to become a positive instrument for living a happier, healthier life.

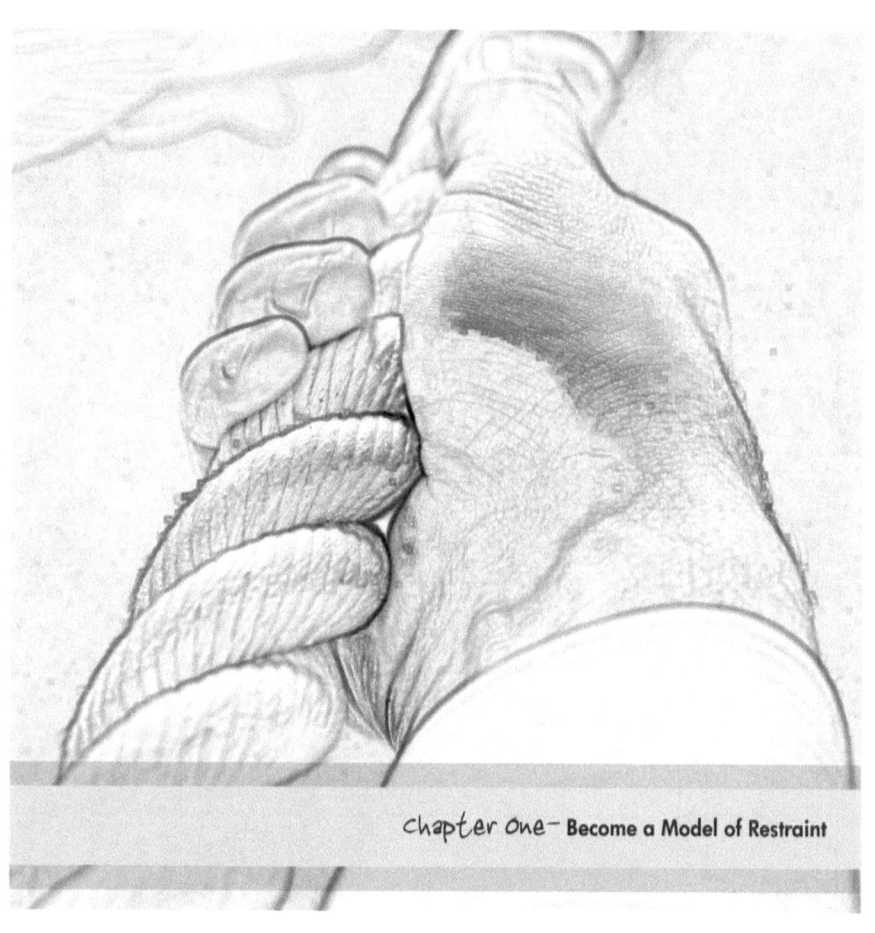

chapter One– Become a Model of Restraint

Chapter One

Become a Model of Restraint

Follow the Success Rules

I truly believe that the best way to avoid the major causes of death, like heart attacks and strokes, is through prevention. Remember that an ounce of prevention is worth a pound of cure. You must assimilate health into our daily living in order to achieve a balanced lifestyle. Remember, discipline is willpower. So you have to become a model of restraint and resist the urge to do whatever is not in alignment with your goal, including restraining how much you eat when trying to lose weight.

For the many years that I have known "Lucky Harry" at my clinic, he has struggled with diabetes and weight control. He is called Lucky Harry because he survived a heart attack.

Lucky Harry considers himself successful because he kept a good job for a very long time. He has been married for thirty-five years to his devoted wife. They have four children who are doing very well. He is flamboyant and often says that he is a happy man, even though he has good and bad days.

His body type would be classified as apple-shaped (as opposed to pear-shaped), which conveys the picture of someone with a lot of excess fat around the belly. Trying to control his weight and diabetes had been his major health dilemmas. The struggle continued, until one more major health risk made his list of problems even longer—a heart attack.

Lucky Harry lost his father to a heart attack when his dad was in his sixties, and Lucky Harry was about the same age. He dreaded the same fate.

Given his history of diabetes, he could develop the so-called silent heart attack mainly because of damage to his nerves. Such a heart attack is very subtle and lacks the dramatic symptom of severe chest pain that may persist for more than fifteen minutes.

Lucky Harry felt sick to his stomach while shoveling snow on the drive way. Then he felt very tired, severe enough for him to abandon what he was doing. He tried to put on a brave face and insisted on just staying home to rest. When his wife noticed that he was gasping for air, she concluded that he was definitely "going downhill," and she made the right decision to call emergency services. He went to the emergency room.

I had just seen Lucky Harry and his wife at my clinic shortly before the heart attack happened, and they were both aware of the downhill rule—a measure of how bad an ailment is. His wife saved his life by quickly assessing his situation. The downhill rule made her not wait any longer at home.

At first, Lucky Harry did not know how to subject his urge of overindulgence to his will. He leaned how to do it using the principles in this book. This couple agreed that my success rules were instrumental in achieving some of their success in dealing with his health challenges.

But are there such things as success rules? Yes. By studying successful people, I discovered that they all had one thing in common: a sense of discipline toward their goals.

I have often believed that success in any of our lives is framed by character traits. They are the anchor that all else emanates from. Discipline is the cornerstone of self-mastery. Self-discipline is the ability to put your desire under the control of your will. In essence, it is self-control. Its basis is the power of the will. And because we make choices using our conscious mind, this quality needs to be internalized if we are to become a magnet for willpower.

Discipline bridges the gap between having knowledge and actually acting on it. It is one thing to make a commitment, but the real test is whether your thinking, behavior, and actions are in alignment with your goals—and whether you stay on the right track after the decision has been made.

Self-discipline has to be directed toward goals. Otherwise it's aimless and unproductive. Goals are the steps that move you toward your purpose, the reason behind doing what you do. Purpose conveys meaning and significance, but goals are the bridge between where you are and where you end up.

The goals have to be clear and specific, so that you can focus or redirect your attention to them. It is easy to say your purpose is better health, but it means very little until you fill in the blanks with what you really want to do in order to achieve your purpose.

Imagine leaving your home without a clear destination! You'd drive around town in circles and then end up nowhere. So why even bother leaving the house without a clear reason for where you are going? It's a waste of time! When you leave home knowing where you are going, it's easy; you just drive straight to where you want to go. Clear goals are important.

Our personal fulfillment comes from achieving the things that we want. Health care is the priority here, but longevity, quality of life, and happiness are also the highly prized key benefits for striving to achieve better health.

Goals should also be balanced. We need harmony between our mind, body, and soul. We want to be strong in those three areas, so we have to build both the intangible inner strength and the physical aspects in order to achieve balance. To identify which of these areas you need to focus on to restore balance in your life, do a self-evaluation by rating yourself on a scale of one to ten in all eight chapters in this book. This will indirectly assess the balance of mind, body, and spirit in your life.

The eight elements that I have presented in the following eight chapters represent the key areas that you need to focus on in order to achieve this balance. Potential goals also flow from these areas, though they are more or less guidelines. The purpose of the outline is to help you focus in creating the goals that are relevant to your needs and, even more importantly, to stimulate you to be disciplined enough to actually do so.

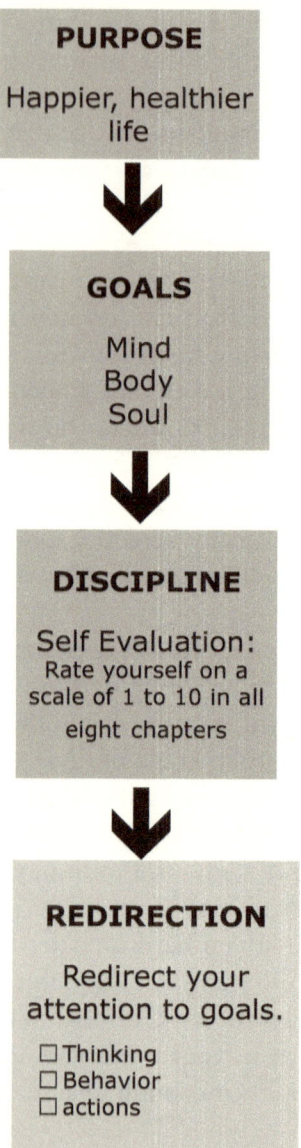

How to Develop a Disciplined Lifestyle

Lucky Harry has often blamed his family tree for his medical woes. He believes that his diabetes, obesity, and heart attack have familial roots. I definitely agree with him, but only to a point. I have often encouraged him to focus on what he could change, because that is where his power lies—learning how to handle the things that he can change. When it comes to weight, there is a set-point that is genetically determined around which most peoples' weight settles. This is a significant factor in weight management and according to different experts may vary from 30 percent to 50 percent.

Lucky Harry's heart attack was a wake-up call. So he decided to stop blaming genetics and do something about his health—to take responsibility for his life. Some people are like him; they wait until something painful happens to them that scares them and moves them out of their comfort zone. And that is when they get out of the little box that they once felt comfortable in, and they try to do something. Contemplating the loss of one's health status could be very scary. This is why fear is such a great motivator.

Lucky Harry was ready for personal growth. The best place to start was self-evaluation. He had to do some sort of reality check. Reality is the difference between what you wish and what is. He wished to have good health, but he had to do something. Just being knowledgeable was not enough.

Lucky Harry had to self-evaluate the eight critical elements for fostering health—the eight secrets of healthy living.

1. Become a Model of Restraint
2. Set Clear Goals
3. Motivate Yourself
4. Apply the downhill rule
5. Obtain Regular Checkups
6. Master Stress
7. Keep Your Ideal Weight
8. Turn Theory into Practice

Lucky Harry reviewed the eight secrets of healthy living at home and measured how disciplined he was. It is easy to do. For each element, he picked out a time period for the activity and assessed how often he stuck to his word. For example, he measured how many times he actually followed his schedule for exercising on the treadmill. He measured how many times each year within the past ten years he'd honored his doctor's appointments for routine checkups. As you may imagine, his scores were between two and four, on a scale of one to ten, when he rated himself.

Lucky Harry turned a corner when he identified an underlying problem: his bitter attitude toward his parents. When he dealt with and rid himself of his bitterness, he could actually start making positive steps toward achieving better health. The baggage was a distraction that was sapping a lot of his energy. This is important, because decisions or choices are made in the mind, and impulse control and judgment are an integral part of the process. Baggage or antagonism means wasted energy.

Self-discipline is the ability to put your desire under the control of your will. In essence, it is self-control. Its basis is the power of the will. This character trait needs to be cultivated and internalized in order to achieve self-mastery. It does not happen automatically.

Another important way of staying disciplined is to learn how to resist the urge to do the things that are not in alignment with your personal goals. Lucky Harry learned how to resist the urge to indulge in eating. And it paid handsomely for cutting down on his calories. That played a major part in his weight loss program. It is a simple habit to alter, but it could make a monumental difference, because the key to losing weight is cutting back on calories and portion sizes.

Discipline starts with a commitment or pledge to stick to a plan of action. We can have the most elaborate plan to get things done, but we must have the discipline to do it to produce results. Results are what counts.

Lucky Harry had a very big gap between his knowledge and action. He had a treadmill in the basement that he got for Christmas many years back. He confided to me that he was held back by procrastination. He kept on saying that he was going to use the machine, but he never got to it. He scored a three on the scale regarding his discipline toward daily exercise. That was less than mediocre, he told me. And he was determined to improve that score with time. He learned that one of the keys to overcoming procrastination is to initiate action, which leads to increased motivation to act.

He is like many people that I speak to as a doctor. Most of them are fine people, very knowledgeable about how to achieve healthy living. The problem is that they do not do it. That leads me to think that knowledge and awareness alone do not move people to action—motivation does!

Fear is arguably the greatest motivator there is. Lucky Harry's heart attack put a lot of fear in him. He was afraid of his health getting worse. He wanted to do anything to stop it. He was worried about not being able to see his grandchildren grow up or enjoy the wealth that he'd worked so hard to accumulate. All these things got him fired up and motivated to act.

One of the things I've often told patients is that spontaneous self-motivation, even though not as strong a motivator as fear, should lead people toward making health a priority. When people wait until something catastrophic happens, like a heart attack, some of the damage has already been done and often cannot be reversed.

Support and encouragement from Harry's wife were also a great source of motivation for him. She bought him a reliable alarm clock to help him get out of bed early in the morning for his exercise. Because of her actions, one of the excuses was pushed out of his list. Slowly Lucky Harry improved on his ability to challenge himself, even when things were tough.

Character Traits

Your ability to succeed in any area of your life, including better health, is framed in your character traits. They give you the anchor on which all else is developed.

Discipline is the key character trait in developing self-mastery. It comes from positive programming of the mind, which means that you constantly match your thoughts, actions, and behaviors with what you want over time. That is how your goals get achieved. Discipline helps you to keep going on a chosen path. That is how things get done. And you reduce the gap between knowledge and action by dwelling on the worthy goals, not distractions. That is what eventually moves you toward the right target.

Positive programming makes you stay focused on the things that are important: for example, the desire to engage in the thoughts, behaviors, and actions that will foster long-term health. This character trait works in concert with other traits, like perseverance, which shares an important similarity with discipline: they are based on willpower. Perseverance is the ability to keep going or trying over and over again. It is very helpful when, although the desire is there, halfway through the run you feel like quitting. Lucky Harry has learned how to use the great force of discipline to align himself with his health goals. This great tool for affecting success is reinforced from within by the need for transformation from negative to positive programming.

Lucky Harry learned how to fill his mind with positive thoughts and images relating to a disciplined lifestyle. He created affirmations that he repeated to himself all day long and shortly before falling asleep. His affirmations would include sayings like "Dessert is just calories" and "I prefer to see those calories in the garbage can rather than on my abdomen." Repeating this affirmation at home when dessert was being served helped him to pass on the sweets more often.

In order to do this he had to subject instant gratification to his volition to what's going to lead to long-term health. Within a month, Lucky Harry changed from a score of three to eight on the scale of one to ten.

He also visualized positive images of success. He liked to see his grandchildren, so he visualized sitting with his grandchildren in impeccable health. As he constantly dwelled on these positive images, they helped raise his level of motivation, and his energy then soared in turn.

Lucky Harry role-played the many other benefits that would come from disciplined action. He imagined himself as a marathon runner finishing a race. He saw himself at the finish line, which gave him a lot of pep as well. That is what helped him go the extra mile on the treadmill.

He also used the law of substitution to thwart impulses that would lead to a negative behavior. This law simply states that you must substitute whatever negative urge you are having with its positive opposite. For example, when Lucky Harry's mouth started to water in anticipation of a sweet treat, he started reviewing the different benefits that he would gain by not eating it. It is like changing a television channel when you do not like what you are seeing (or thinking)—you do not try to fight with it; you simply change the channel. The mind works best that way. That is how you move your attention from what you do not like to what you want.

So Lucky Harry would say things like, "Dessert is just calories!" And yes, he is right—it's just calories. He said to himself, "I would prefer to have my diabetes and weight under control. That will give me longevity and great quality of life."

Positive programming eventually leads to the formation of a desired habit. This is because your reasoning mind engages your subconscious mind, which is the seat of long-term memory, and through repetition a habit is formed. The activity or action in question becomes a routine. That is how it becomes assimilated as a lifestyle. At this point, doing that questionable activity is not a choice anymore. Freedom from it could really be enjoyable.

Impulse control is the key to discipline. In order to achieve this, you must be hungry for expanding self-discipline. Positive programming then happens; otherwise it withers and dies. It is easy to resist the urge to do what's not in alignment with your goals when you use of the law of substitution—simply change the channel!

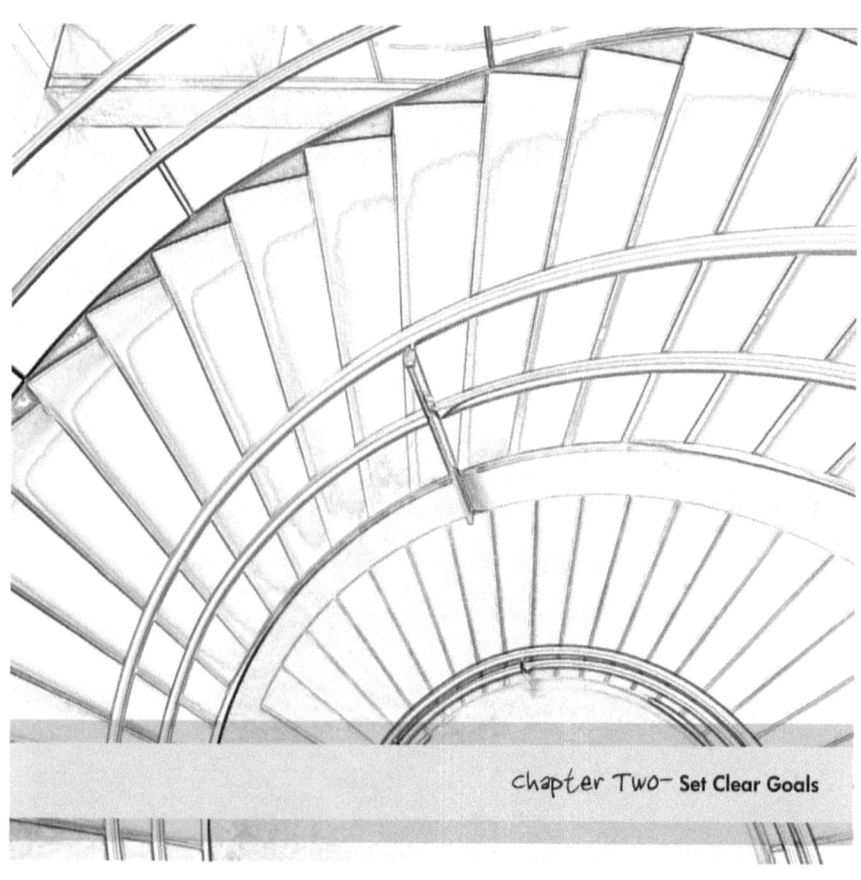

chapter Two– **Set Clear Goals**

Chapter Two

Set Clear Goals

Lucky Harry represents a very complex medical case because he has diabetes and has had a heart attack, as well as trouble with weight control. I had to help him figure out his profile and the corresponding diet regimen he needed to be on.

He was very frustrated because he had tried many different diets, but nothing helped. Instead, his weight increased. His blood sugar levels were all over the map. He had been recovering from a heart attack and lost six weeks of work. Despite these problems, he had neither a solid plan to improve his situation nor any goals. His description of what he was doing was very vague.

Lucky Harry still had an apple-shaped body, meaning that his weight was carried in the midsection of his body. This weight distribution is associated with certain pathologies, such as heart disease and gall bladder stones. Just looking at him, I knew that he needed a major lifestyle change in order to reverse some of his pathology. Before I helped him figure out his profile and his needs, I had to explain why clear goals and a plan were necessary to succeed.

Some people do not think about this, but a good deal of our lives revolve around challenging our mind with what we want. These are thought impulses, and the end result is either to sustain our attention or redirect it to make a goal happen through our thoughts, behaviors, and actions. That is why it is important to dwell on or present what you want to your mind. It will then match your thinking, behaviors and actions to get it. That is why goals are important. They tell your mind where you're going. That is why being goal-directed keeps you on track

You cannot shoot a target without seeing it. Think about a laser beam. It has many medical applications, but it is simply a beam of light that is concentrated and put into focus. That is what goals do. They bring your whole person into focus. They also stimulate and energize you, especially when they are big enough to get the adrenaline running through your body, making your heart thump. They also have to be clear enough. Otherwise you cannot reach a specific target.

Lucky Harry was very vague in his description of what he was doing. He had no overall purpose that acted as a thread to hold everything together. When I met with him, he decided to make healthy living a priority. His purpose was to become the healthiest person he could be. So he set a standard, important because he could then keep pushing the envelope to get better and better, which is very stimulating. It brings simple activities from the head to the heart, creating passion.

The wider purpose gives significance and meaning. It makes you feel fulfilled with or about its attainment. But you need small action steps on a daily basis to move you toward the target. The purpose is more a long-term goal. The goals and the sub-goals are the things that move you forward to achieve your purpose.

I told Lucky Harry that his goals had to be communicated in simple words or phrases. They did not have to be long. These actions steps had to be assimilated into his lifestyle in order to be effective. Lucky Harry's action steps included understanding that:

- Physical fitness begins in the mind with the spark of desire.
- Physical begins with mental fitness.
- He must limit his food intake by drinking water before each meal.
- Food is medicine, and he must eat a balanced diet of protein, carbohydrates, and fat.
- He must make meals at home and avoid processed and packaged foods, as they are filled with sugar, salt, and unhealthy fats.

Also, clear and specific goals help pace peoples' lives. Otherwise they just waste their energy on aimless activities. When you think about it, our minds control our ability to organize and plan what we want to do. It helps us put our thoughts, behaviors, and actions together. We form habits when our minds are preoccupied with specific goals. The repetition from our reasoning mind eventually causes the subconscious mind to make it second nature.[1]

The best way to set goals for your health needs is to first do clinical profiling. You must first figure out what your issues are. This is very simple. It could be that you want to lose weight. It could also be because you have diabetes and want to have it under control. Cardiac rehabilitation (as is the case after a heart attack) could be the motivation. Lucky Harry was unfortunate to have all of these conditions, so his clinical profile was very complex. Despite that fact, I was able to help him simplify it. If you can understand Lucky Harry's clinical profile, then you can easily figure out your own. I will use weight control as an illustration because it is a very common health problem.

You do not have to wait until you are overweight before you start working on your weight. Be proactive. It is easier to maintain your weight than to wait until you become overweight before you do something about it. This applies not only to weight management; it applies to everything that contributes to a healthy life.

Live as if you have the common risk factors that increase your susceptibility to diseases like heart attack, stroke, anxiety, and diabetes. I find that it is the best way to ward them off. Why? Because some conditions, like strokes, can leave you with irreversible complications, like paralysis of your limbs, that can put you in a wheelchair for the rest of your life. So here is my point—if you wait until you have a stroke or heart attack before you start watching your diet or modify your lifestyle, then it is sometimes too late to act. The cholesterol would have already done the damage as it is deposited on your arteries. It becomes almost impossible to reverse the process.

Being overweight or unfit increases your risk for these common diseases. Heart attacks can be fatal; they are responsible for about 50 percent of deaths in North America alone.[2] Make your weight-loss goal clear and specific. For example, say to yourself, "I will lose five pounds this month, and I will exercise half an hour on a daily basis." In general, a Body Mass Index (BMI), a universal standard for assessing ideal weight, of less than 25 is considered normal. Being overweight refers to a BMI from 25 to 29.9 kg/m, and obesity refers to a BMI of more than 30. You can work

---

1   Amen, Dr. Daniel. *Change Your Brain, Change Your Life: The Breakthrough Program for Conquering Anxiety, Depression, Obsessiveness, Anger, and Impulsiveness.* Three Rivers Press. 1999.

2

out your ideal weight using the BMI chart in Chapter Seven, or you can use your waist size to keep track of how you are doing.

Following a healthy lifestyle wards off most of these common killers. It has been shown that even a 10-pound weight loss will lead to a significant drop in your risk for these conditions.[3]

No matter your clinical profile, you can match yourself to one of the four diet regimens discussed below. If you want to eat in such a way as to prevent diabetes, control your weight, and ward off heart attacks, then eat like the new Lucky Harry. He belongs to the Balanced Diet regimen.

The Four Diet Regimens

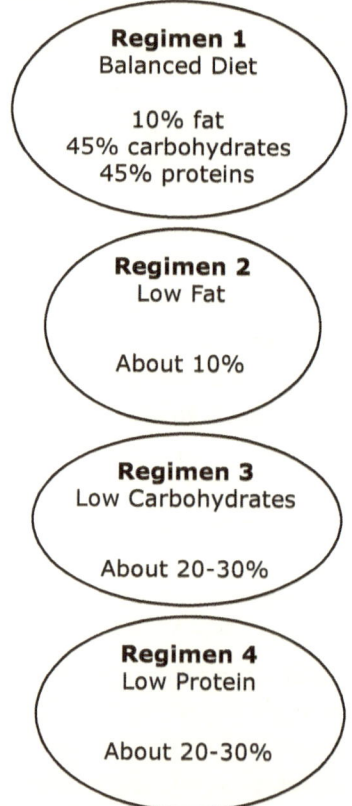

Regimen 1: Balanced Diet

The essence of Regimen 1, called the balanced diet, is about 10 percent

3   Tallia, Alfred F., Dennis A. Cardone, Kenneth H. Ibsen, and David F. Howarth. *Swanson's Family Practice Review: A Problem-Oriented Approach*, Fifth Edition. Mosby. 2004.

fat, 45 percent carbohydrates, and 45 percent proteins. It is generally one that respects the suggested proportions of food groups above. It is a diet like most—high in fruits and vegetables and low in fat. There is significant crossover between the different regimens, but all are appropriate for those who seek a balanced lifestyle to prevent the major killers like obesity, heart attacks, diabetes, stroke, and high blood pressure. So the 50 percent of the population that is fit and does not need to lose weight belongs here too. If you have the risk factors that make you a strong candidate for a particular diet regimen, then stick to it. That is, you may be healthy, but if heart disease, diabetes, high blood pressure, or stroke run in your family, your odds are higher than the average person.

Regimen 2: Low Fat

The focus here is to keep the fat extremely low ($\geq$ 10 percent). The types of people who will benefit most from this regimen are those who have had a heart attack, stroke, or any severe cardiovascular pathology. It is questionable as to whether plaque on the arteries can be reversed. However, you need to be more aggressive in limiting the amount of fat in your diet because there is already a lot of plaque deposition and stiffening of the arteries. Fats stimulate the gall bladder to eliminate the enzyme that digests fat. The gall bladder then contracts following the stimulation, leading to pain in the abdomen. Also, people with risk factors for gall bladder disease will do well with this diet. A clue could be an apple-shaped body, which means carrying weight around the midsection.

Regimen 3: Low Carbohydrates

The focus here is low carbohydrates (20 to 30 percent). The rationale here is that your pancreas is already having difficulty dealing with sugars, so you do not need to further strain it with more than a necessary amount of carbohydrates. Even more important are the complex carbohydrates that come from grain products and fruits and vegetables. Compared to the simple sugars like glucose (found in table sugar), the complex carbohydrates get digested and absorbed much more slowly from the gut into the bloodstream. In that way they do not make your blood sugar level swing to a quick high. That means your blood sugars will be kept a little more stable. That is key in controlling diabetes and avoiding dangerous fluctuations that may easily lead to low blood sugar (hypoglycemia).

Regimen 4: Low Protein

The focus here is low protein (20 to 30 percent). The people who will get the most benefit are those with certain kidney problems, when their kidneys are having trouble eliminating protein waste. Note that there are certain kidney pathologies where you may instead need more proteins, like protein shakes, because your kidneys are losing lots of protein. Get your health care provider to help you determine where you belong, if it is not clear. There are also certain bowel pathologies like celiac disease where difficulty in absorption of proteins may lead to swelling in your legs due to lack of proteins. Also, those with celiac disease may need more proteins in their diet, not less.

What does it all mean?

With the balanced diet, the goal is to prevent plaque formation, which predisposes people to heart attack and strokes. Weight control and diabetes management are also considered. Fat intake should be 10 percent, complex carbohydrates about 45 percent, and protein about 45 percent too. The key to weight loss is the balance between calories taken in and those expended. So cutting down on portion sizes is crucial. But there is an important chemical balance here between carbohydrates and proteins. A ratio of about 50:50 is optimal.[4] The reason is that carbohydrates make your body secrete insulin and store fat, and they make you crave more sugars. This leads to the "sugar blues," where you feel very tired a few hours after a high-carbohydrate meal.

On the other hand, proteins make your body secrete glucagon, which modulates the effect of insulin and makes your body burn more fat. That leads to weight control, of course!

It has been shown that the diet that reverses plaque is 70 percent complex carbohydrates, 20 percent protein, and 10 percent fat.[5] This is easy to say theoretically, but the problem is that once the arteries have been coated with plaque, it becomes very difficult to reverse the process of degeneration.

If you are having difficulty understanding the diet regimens or trouble with managing your weight, contact a health care provider to determine

---

4   Sears, Dr. Barry. *The Zone: A Dietary Road Map to Lose Weight Permanently: Reset Your Genetic Code: Prevent Disease: Achieve Maximum Physical Performance.* Regan Books. 1995.

5   Oz, Dr. Mehmet, Michael Dr. Roizen. *You: On a Diet: The Insider's Guide to Easy and Permanent Weight Loss.* Thorsons/Element. 2010.

your specific dietary needs. Also check for possible secondary medical problems.

The key to weight control is the calories-in and calories-out balance. But where your calories come from is important. That is why you need to first do your clinical profile in order to determine which kind of diet is most suitable for you. You can either go by what medical problems you have or those you are prone to get.

When blood sugar rises too fast, a lot of insulin is put into the bloodstream by the pancreas, which may produce a quick drop in blood sugar, leading to hypoglycemia (very low sugar),often about two to three hours following a meal including big quantities of carbohydrates, especially those with high glycemic indices. Because it contains simple sugars like glucose that are quickly absorbed from the gut into the bloodstream, table sugar is not good.

Even amongst complex carbohydrates, those with a much lower glycemic index are better because their rate of absorption into the bloodstream is slow, which prevents blood sugar from spiking. That puts brakes on the hunger mechanism that I will explain in Chapter Seven. And the advantages are many. You do not feel hunger pangs, so you do not eat ravenously and add lots of calories. The sugar blues are avoided, which staves off the fatigue that is associated with the low blood sugar that goes with it. And less fluctuation in blood sugar levels means more smooth control of and/or prevention of diabetes.

Learn more about the glycemic indices of complex carbohydrates. Potatoes have a very high glycemic index, so try to avoid eating them in large quantities.

The fourth diet regimen is one with low proteins. Quite often protein could represent about 20 to 30 percent of your diet. There are situations where this could be applicable, as for someone who has severe kidney damage, where the kidney cannot deal with high protein loads. Reducing the amount of protein means the kidneys don't have to deal with a large protein load.

But there are people who may also need high proteins. For example, their kidney pathology could mean that they are losing proteins through urine, so they may instead need more. Extreme malnutrition with minimal protein consumption, or bowel pathology, or surgical stomach bypass surgery for weight control may lead to the need for a high-protein diet. Some protein shakes provide high amounts of protein. Proteins help fluid stay in the bloodstream. Some people have swelling in their legs due to a lack of protein.

If you are in doubt about your clinical profile and the appropriate diet regimen, contact a health care professional. Your doctor or dietician will offer great counsel and may sometimes need to do testing to figure out what is best for you.

To put health promotion into perspective, it has been my experience as a physician that the majority of amputations and kidney dialysis are is due to diabetes, and that 90 percent of diabetic cases are Type II, largely due to a sedentary, stressed lifestyle with poor food choices. Notice the domino effect here.

You can clearly see why an ounce of prevention is truly worth a pound of cure. There are definitely monumental challenges to inspiring and encouraging people to be more disciplined or even harder, to change their lifestyles. Hard as it is may be, we cannot give up, because with repetition, we hope that the "light bulb" eventually turns on!

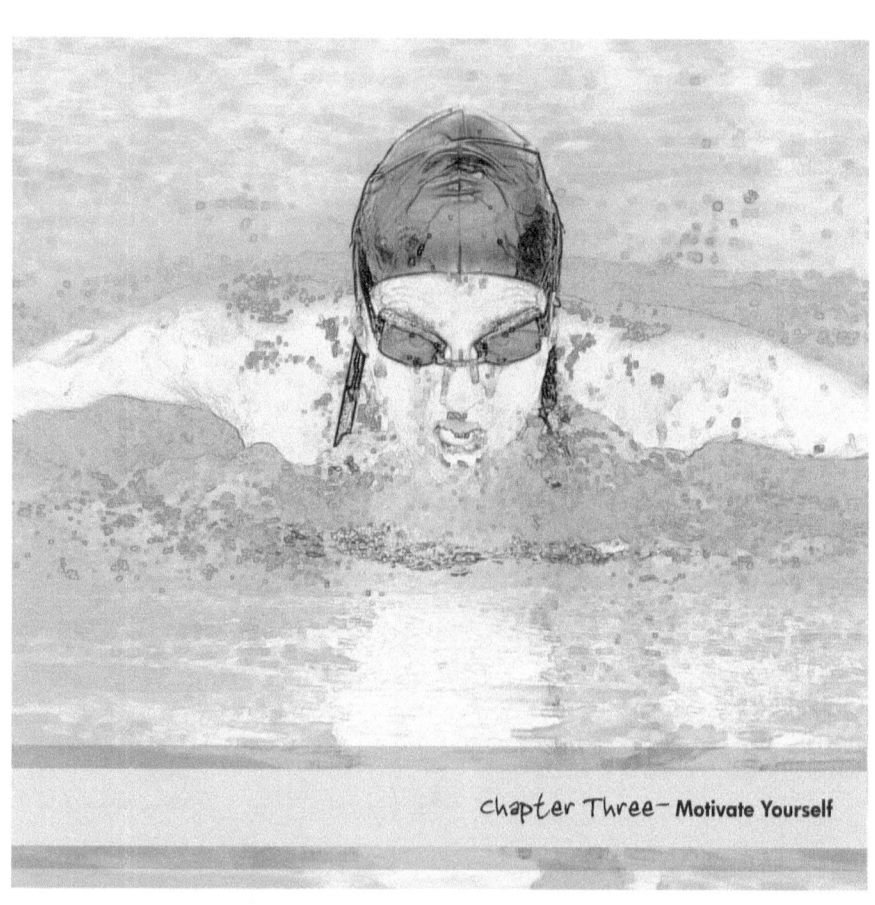
Chapter Three— Motivate Yourself

Chapter Three:

Motivate Yourself

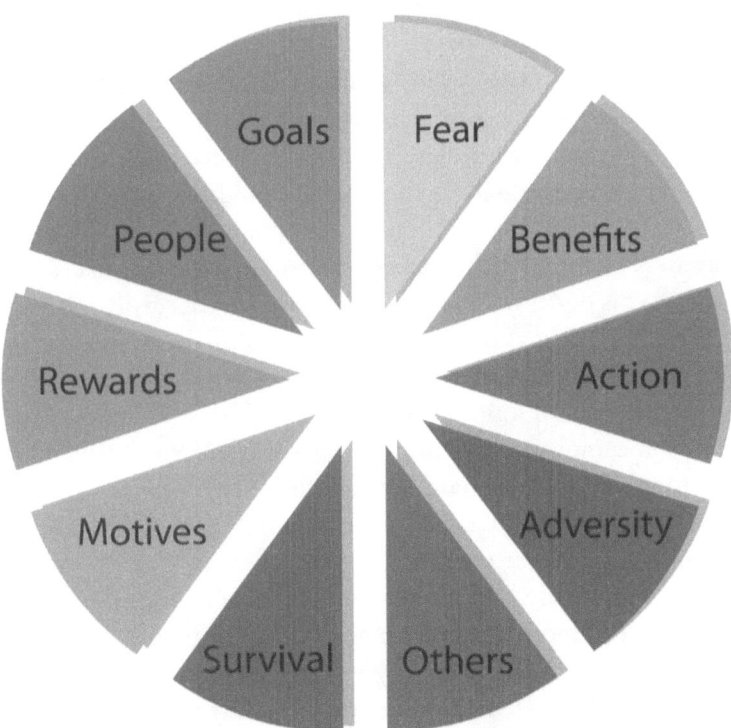

Figure 1: Motivation Wheel

What Determines Motivation?

Lucky Harry had his goals written on paper. His next hurdle was to jumpstart his action plan for healthy living. In order to become decisive, he had to break his cycle of procrastination. That needed a lot of motivation.

According to Brian Tracy, author and motivational speaker, fear is the most powerful motivator, especially the fear of losing what one already has: good health, in this case. As you can see on the Motivation Wheel (Figure 1), there are many other factors that determine motivation.

Lucky Harry had difficulties managing his weight and diabetes. But he still thought that he had good health until the heart attack hit. It served as his wake-up call. It scared him, especially because his father had died from a heart attack some years back. It was a great source of motivation for his total health makeover.

There are two kinds of motivation: extrinsic and intrinsic. Extrinsic motivation comes from the outside, either from other people or through rewards. In contrast, intrinsic motivation comes from within.

Each person carries within them what could be the perfect source of incentive for doing whatever they love to do. The essence is to increase our awareness of some of the factors that may move us to action. But to cooperate in this endeavor, our reasoning mind, especially the prefrontal area of the brain, is key; because it is the area of the mind that helps us focus on what we want.[6] Our subconscious mind aids in the process, because it is the seat of long-term memory and habit formation.

To become motivated, stimulate this part of the mind by paying attention to your goals. We have to help our brain cooperate in the process of success. It is not enough just to write our goals down. We have to act on them in order to produce results.

Lucky Harry's wife told me that moving the treadmill around in the basement was the most exercise he got from it. The treadmill had been a great Christmas gift. He was very excited about it and went on a daily exercise spree for one week, and then did virtually nothing for a year. She said that the dust on the treadmill could fill a garbage can.

So the key was to get Lucky Harry to connect his goals with his imagination. He created goals according to his needs. But having them hanging on the wall in the basement did him no good. He had to bring

---

6   Amen, Dr. Daniel. *Change Your Brain, Change Your Life: The Breakthrough Program for Conquering Anxiety, Depression, Obsessiveness, Anger, and Impulsiveness.* Three Rivers Press. 1999.

his goals up from the basement to his desk so that he could challenge his mind with them all the time.

This process is called *emotionalization*; we make the connection between our brain and our heart. That is how we become passionate about our goals or dreams.

Another thing that he did was create a blueprint from the goals by making affirmations. Affirmations are short, positive statements that are easy to remember. He repeated the affirmations with conviction as many times as possible throughout the day, especially shortly before falling asleep to involve the subconscious mind, which is very powerful shortly before falling asleep and shortly after waking up.[7] That is how we redirect our attention to what we want.

So first he wrote down his affirmations. That was how he initiated them. But in order to create them, his imagination had to get involved. He told his mind what he wanted by repeating the affirmations. That lead to daily renewal in his belief in his goals. As the subconscious mind implants affirmations, it becomes a second-nature routine.

And so Lucky Harry reinforced his can-do attitude. He changed his internal dialogue to pay attention to the goals that he set for himself. Those were the things that his mind dwelled on, and that is what he wanted.

Lucky Harry's score on the eight elements for achieving a healthy lifestyle was less than mediocre. His aim was to get on track and stay motivated enough to keep doing the things that were important. Renewing his belief on a daily basis by looking in the mirror and vocalizing his goals to himself became a very powerful force for willing what he wanted into his imagination. It put him in touch with his basic impulses. That is why belief in your purpose or goals inspires becoming connected with them.

That was how Lucky Harry's thoughts, behaviors, and actions were modeled to move him toward his desired target. I told him to see himself as if he had already accomplished his goals. Imagining a happy ending is very motivating. He thought of himself as a marathon runner finishing his race. When he went to bed at night, he visualized himself at the end of his run on the treadmill. He said to himself all day long, "I am becoming fit," and "I can change my life if I change my thoughts." His affirmations were written both in the present tense and in the first person.

There is never a conflict between the reasoning mind and the subconscious mind when we match our actions with our desires, because

7   Nkut, Dr. Alfred. *Leadership For Success: A Dynamic Model of Influence.* AuthorHouse. 2010

the subconscious does what the command center of the brain wills it to do. Telling the mind that you are fit gives it a positive message, which is more powerful for making a positive change than a negative one. Knowing that, we must choose to stick to positive messages. Psychologically and physiologically, being positive is better and moves us forward.

Yes! Our perception influences our chemistry! A positive message is more uplifting and leads to more excitement. That makes your energy and motivation soar. Ambitious goals are also motivating. What you are doing is redirecting your attention to what you want. That is how you become a channel for what you want. That is how you program your mind to bring what you want to experience to pass. Your mind brings the factors that you need to achieve those goals, whether it is motivation from within or people and circumstances that will make your goal happen.

The great psychologist James Allen made the point that the aim that you cherish in your soul is what you will live your life by and what you will become.[8]

People are also very important in motivating us to achieve what we want. Lucky Harry was very highly influenced by his wife. She saved his life by encouraging him to go to the emergency room at the hospital when he was having his heart attack. She also took the initiative to buy him a good alarm clock to get him up each morning to exercise. She also made him feel guilty about eating dessert after dinner. Lucky Harry tried to pass on dessert most of the time. He had never gotten that far before. He was more mindful of what he put in his mouth. He was living consciously.

He considered the motive behind why he put food in his mind. So he started using food as a medicine, not entertainment. He stopped using comfort food. He used to get out of bed in the night and indulge with a big bowl of chocolate. So when that thought came to mind, he reminded himself that a bowl of sweets was just calories that would increase his weight and make his diabetes harder to manage. So he played the benefits of passing on dessert, and it worked!

People can influence us in many other ways. Sometimes just sticking around people who are disciplined in doing what we want to do is important. Lucky Harry followed his wife's example of passing on dessert. Each time he did it, his wife put a coin in a jar for him to reward him later with something better. She never got around to sharing with me what it was that she bought for Lucky Harry using the coins she saved. But the big grin on his face made me understand that it was something great!

---

8   Allen, James. *As a Man Thinketh*. CreateSpace. 2010

Doing something together, especially for the same reasons, is very stimulating. That is why exercising in a group is much less boring. People sometimes even hire a health coach to help them. Simply indirectly forcing you to place your activities within a routine is helpful. Lucky Harry's wife was very dedicated to seeing him become healthy, so she bought him a dog to help him pace himself. He had to get up early enough to let the dog out. He had to take him out for exercise. And indirectly his routine was established.

There are two ways to respond to adversity. You either shrink back or expand. Lucky Harry, with enormous pressure from his wife, chose to evolve. Adversity pushes people out of their comfort zone. They lose the false security and then take a risk without fear of failure. They realize that they have got nothing to lose!

Lucky Harry was very fearful of a heart attack, so when it happened, he did not play the victim and feel sorry for himself. He used it to great effect. He used it to build both his character and his hope. The event increased his inner strength, which correlates with a higher level of motivation. Why? Well, when you lose your get-up-and-go attitude, whatever the reason, it becomes difficult to get excited about things. The low energy, or vitality, correlates with boredom and low motivation.

Another important advantage of adversity is that it builds perseverance. That little toughness that we gain from a mishap makes us see a speed bump as an opportunity to rest, not stop. People who do not possess the quality of perseverance look at a speed bump as a stop sign. They stop. That is the wrong thing to do.

You can look for a significant other to motivate you, or you can lead yourself to accomplish the things that you want. Again, remember that the greater part of motivation is intrinsic—it comes from within. So use it. Cultivate it. Otherwise you let it wither. I believe that there is an amount of this quality that is inborn and another part that comes from learning how to move ourselves to action; still another part comes from rewards that incentivize us.

If you are an early riser, like me, start your day with your priorities. I think that the reason is obvious. We possess only a finite amount of energy, and at the beginning of the day we have a little more, so use it for the things that matter most. If you prize your health, then starting your day with an activity that will better your health is crucial and will move you on the track toward your goal of healthy living.

But you can start with the unpleasant activities for the same reason—you have a bigger store of energy at the beginning of the day. So let your late-day activities be the ones that you seem to naturally love. Why? Because it is easier to be motivated doing the things that you like. Another reality is that we should take responsibility for doing even the things that we do not like. And even if you do not like to exercise on a daily basis, you have to because it is important for keeping healthy.

But here is how you trick your mind. Rather than think about the exercise, saturate your mind with the benefits of doing it. That will give you more incentive. The expression, "Fake it until you feel it" soon becomes true. And at that time, exercise is not a chore anymore. That is when you identify with exercise! It becomes part of your image. That is how you bring yourself to feeling motivated when you think of exercise or any other activity for fostering healthy living.

So, in order to stay motivated, you must internalize as many of the determinants as possible. Saturate your mind with them. I truly believe that seeing yourself with the "prize" sustains hope for success.

Act with Passion

Lucky Harry came to realize that the reason he was still overweight was because he had not made up his mind to be thin and fit. Many limiting beliefs were keeping him behind. He thought that he was too big to exercise and that he inherited his apple shape from his father. And he believed strongly that there was nothing he could do about it. It took his wife and me many attempts to convince him that there was a certain percentage that he could work to try and change. It was those things that he *could* change that were important.

Belief is so important in our effort to become what we think. When we constantly think of the things that we believe in, that is how the belief process happens. We present what we want to our imagination, maybe in the form of goals, in order to form a mental picture of it. That is how we will it and create it.

The connection between belief and creating, the so-called *placebo effect*, has been well studied and observed anecdotally as well. Here is how it works.

One group of people in pain, let's call them Group A, are given an injection or pill of something benign (having no actually positive or negative effect on them). Another group of people in pain, let's call them Group B, are given an injection or pill with a pain reliever (such as morphine). Both groups were blindfolded so they did not know what they were being given. It was found that 30 percent of the people in Group A, who were not given any pain reliever, reported feeling less pain.[9]

The reason that 30 percent of Group A reported less pain even though they were given a placebo is because the belief in the placebo stimulates the brain to secrete endorphins, which have the same pain relieving effects in the body as the medication does. What this means is that positive belief is very powerful, and that it can change our chemistry and physiology.

A lot of people are like Lucky Harry. They possess very limiting beliefs that hold them back. Sometimes people know that their behavior is irrational, yet they still continue to do it.

Recently I spoke to a young man who has been smoking for a long time. He was seeing me because he was having trouble breathing. He knew all the problems that he could get from smoking, yet it did not stop him from doing it. Like most people who deal with substance abuse problems, he believed that he needed it in order to feel good. Rather than take personal responsibility, he blamed the addiction.

Surely, part of substance abuse and dependency comes from the false belief that the substance is needed in order to feel good or get through the day. This "lack" mentality creates an emptiness within that justifies the need for an external source in order to be happy.[10] The individual keeps reaching out for more substance in order to feel happy. This young man at least took some responsibility by acknowledging that he did it for the joy of it and also to bring down his stress level. But I pointed out to him that in theory that could be true, but practically not being able to breathe would cause him more than just stress—it was costing him his health! Peer pressure was part of his problem; he said that his wife was very controlling and smoked too. So trying to fit in was one of his motives.

I also saw one fellow who was constantly developing infections in his arm because he was injecting himself with street drugs. His mother

9   Placebo. Wikipedia. 27 July 2010. <http://en.wikipedia.org/wiki/Placebo>

10   Nkut, Dr. Alfred. *Leadership For Success: A Dynamic Model of Influence.* AuthorHouse. 2010.

was aware of the fact that this fellow's partner had hepatitis C infection, which could be deadly. She tried to reason with him to stop using the same needles that his partner was using. And he refused. Irrational, but real. Fear of rejection has often been cited as the reason why someone would want to follow the crowd and not do what is right. But this is, in my opinion, ignoring personal responsibility. Note that is has been shown that uncontrolled behavior that feeds the vicious cycle of addiction could also partly be due to damage to certain parts of the brain, notably, the frontal area.[11]

So Lucky Harry left his limiting beliefs behind him. That is a very important in moving forward. He then became goal-oriented. He established health goals to achieve. He was instructed on how to use his imagination to will his goal. He repeated the affirmations to himself all day long with confidence and passion. Getting him to emotionalize his goals was a very important step. He had to act the way he wanted to feel. In order to feel motivated, you have to act with determination and passion.

William James, one of the early American psychologists, observed: Actions follow thoughts and feelings follow actions. This makes sense; emotions are impulses of energy that follow thoughts, actions, and behaviors or experiences.

---

11   Amen, Dr. Daniel. *Change Your Brain, Change Your Life: The Breakthrough Program for Conquering Anxiety, Depression, Obsessiveness, Anger, and Impulsiveness.* Three Rivers Press. 1999.

The diagram below shows how actions can lead to motivation and then to further action.

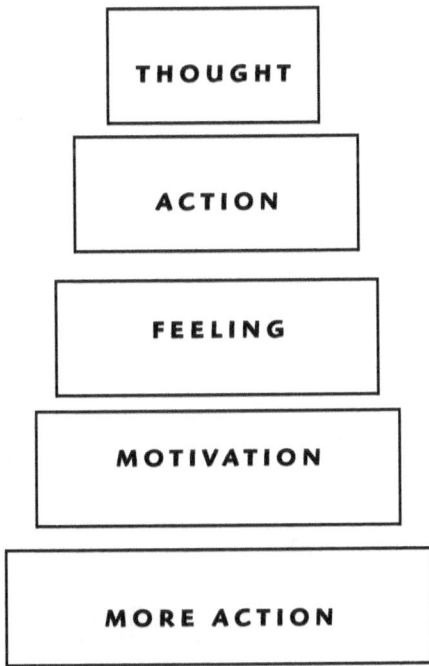

So, the more you do, the more you feel like doing, but the thought must come first.

To help overcome his procrastination, Lucky Harry was told to force himself to get out of bed and exercise in the morning, whether he was in the mood or not. His bad habit had delayed him from taking action or making important decisions. With passion, he repeated his affirmations immediately to himself: "I am the sole architect of my life experience," and "I can do it for my wife and grandchildren." That helped him to take his first action step. Once he overcame the procrastination, he initiated an action, and the energy created a momentum that only kept growing with additional action. Harry's smile and the spring he put in his step were very stimulating to his brain, firing him up for immediate action.

Sometimes setting a start date for taking the first step also helps put pressure on people to act if they are not ready to act just yet.

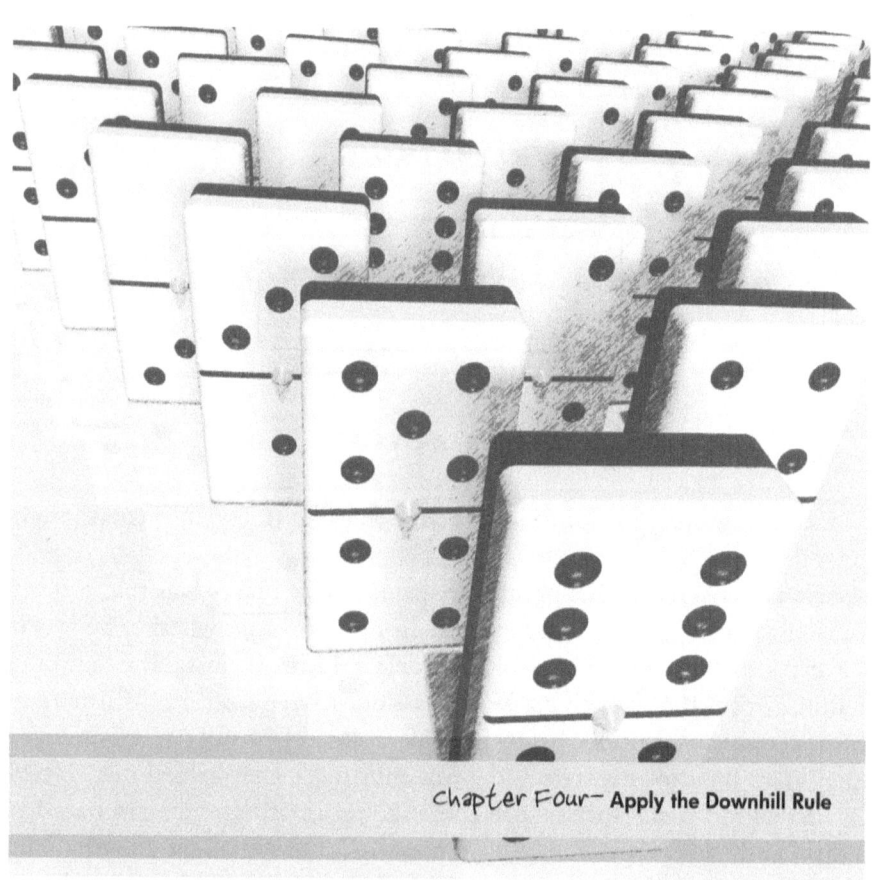

chapter Four— **Apply the Downhill Rule**

Chapter Four

Apply the Downhill Rule

Learning to assess the severity of any medical condition is important. Earlier, I explained how Lucky Harry's wife saved his life using the downhill rule, an index that measures how serious an ailment is, which is important when deciding when an expert opinion is necessary. Most people know that the right setting for treating a heart attack is the emergency room, and they call their local emergency response system. The question most people wonder about, I think, is when to use the emergency system. This is where the client's link to the system is crucial.

I sign insurance forms on a daily basis for people to get paid by their insurance companies for lost time at work. Most of the time it is because of very common things, like a viral illness. So knowing how to use the downhill rule tool will save time and money for everyone. In this chapter I will show you how to use the downhill rule, employing a viral illness as an example. Most people have either had a cold or seen someone with a cold. Each day, I see many people come into my clinic with just a cough.

Most people know about viral illnesses, and that they will pass. Only a few lead to complications that a doctor needs to assess. Making a connection with a telephone advisory option, a pharmacist, or a clinic in a timely and appropriate manner can ease the pressure on medical resources.

If you understand how to apply the downhill rule to a cold, you can use the insight to assess any number of medical problems. It is an indirect assessment of the impact of the problem, which is an important step in knowing what course of action to take.

Each day at my medical clinic, I see many people come in with only a cough. Indirectly assessing the impact of their cough on their sleep tells me whether they need cough medicine or not. Imagine how much cough medicine I would be prescribing if I did not first assess the impact of a person's cough on their life! Simple, but it works.

Last year, at the peak of the flu season, health helplines became jammed. Quite often I see people at my clinic who waited for hours on the telephone before speaking to a medical professional. Sometimes they waited for so long that they got frustrated and then quit.

Someone who saw me was very upset because he waited on the phone for a very long time. This person had a terminal kidney problem, had not passed urine for a day, and, as you can imagine, had almost unbearable abdominal pain, due to the pressure from urine retention. If this person had any understanding of the downhill rule, he wouldn't have been waiting on the phone to be told what he should have already known—go to the emergency room!

I remember a frustrated parent who said that she waited on the phone for very long, only to be told to put a Band-Aid on the bruise on her daughter's face. She concluded that the solution offered by the health professional on the phone was an insult to her intelligence. I wondered loudly why she thought as much. She said that she had been worried about a concussion all day long. She was not exactly a model of restraint; she wanted me to order a head scan. I did my best to explain to her that my clinical judgment, especially when combined with the downhill rule, was more than enough to deal with the situation. Also, the severity of an injury to the head is important but not always the key, because seemingly minute head injuries, even those without a large bump, can cause severe brain damage. But even with very little experience, a serious head injury or concussion is easy to diagnose when symptoms appear hours later. There is not much medical professionals can do except educate parents to watch for the symptoms. When there is true brain damage, any combination of symptoms, depending on the severity, may be evident. Headaches, vomiting, dizziness, and confusion are the most common ones. It's almost impossible to have these symptoms and be smiling at the same time!

Telephone health helplines have their limitations; sometimes it is not easy to put the medical situation in context over the phone. When someone walks in to the exam room smiling and looking focused, it is obvious that he doesn't have a concussion. But how could one make this kind of assessment on the phone? The hysterical parent with tears rolling down her cheeks may sorely need empathy, which may be a bit difficult to give through the phone as well. Medicine is not an exact science, and sometimes it's almost impossible to resolve some of these issues on the phone.

But solutions may sometimes seem so simple that you wonder why you even went to see a doctor, had common sense prevailed. Consider a ten-year-old boy with a cough, fever, runny nose, headache, and diarrhea. Initially, the kinds of things that would come to mind include a viral illness like the common cold or flu, bacterial infection, or superinfection. These are the kinds of problems that I anticipate that he may get according to his presentation. So those are the things that I will look for both in my case history and examination. That will guide me to ask the right questions in my history and know what to look for in the examination.

We dig for gold only where we expect to find some. Otherwise we dig all over the place, and that is not effective. Knowing how to use the downhill rule will significantly reduce how many people end up seeing a doctor unnecessarily. Why? Because most of the people with the above symptoms or a reasonable similar combination of symptoms do not really need to see a doctor. They are probably having a viral illness of some sort, which is, by nature, self-limiting. It means that they will get well with time, with the exception of the minority of cases that were initially bacterial or viral illnesses that later became superinfections, which is how a viral illness kills most of the time. At first, the virus invades your body, weakening your body and immune system, opening the door to being attacked by bacteria.

The lungs may get easily infected, leading to a double pneumonia, typically by the staphylococcus strain. Double pneumonia means a viral and bacterial pneumonia occur together.

When one or more of these criteria is present, we know this boy is going downhill:

- He feels that he is getting worse.
- He is not sleeping well.
- His fever does not break after three days.
- He is not eating or drinking well.
- He looks sick or gloomy.

The above downhill rule criteria are meant to complement your thinking process in determining how bad an ailment is. I suggest that you consider that you are getting worse when one or more of these criteria is present. The reason is to make you very sensitive to your situation, not in the way of causing undue hysteria, but to aid you in making a timely decision.

The five main benefits of using the downhill rule are:

1. Minimize time lost from work due to illness.
2. Reduce the pressure on pharmacists and doctors.
3. Reduce crowding in clinics and hospital emergency rooms.
4. Reduce jamming telephone health helplines.
5. Save money at all levels, including insurance and technical infrastructure

The essence of this rule is to help you follow the best course of action for your ailment. But even in the worst of situations, staying calm and focused is your first rule because you cannot make reasonable decisions once you are confused. Should that happen, the voice of reason should prevail. That may mean picking up the phone and making the "intuitive" call. Hysteria is never advisable because the anxiety and stress generated from it just feeds into whatever problem you or the ill person has.

You definitely do not want to wait for too long before you act, if you do have to act. And it is often better to ask not only questions but the right ones, especially when you are not sure of what to do. I think that just being aware of the downhill rule puts you ahead of the pack, allowing you to deal with your problem in a more or less expedient manner.

Another reason for increasing awareness is to be on the safe side. There is a fine line, as you can imagine, for acting promptly in such a way as to avoid either being too late to act or inciting hysteria. I think that timely action would avoid hysteria down the road.

Accurate use of the downhill rule also depends on how intuitive and confident you are.

You can see why knowing whether your medical problem is getting worse or better is very important. I am sure that you have been asked these simple questions before by a doctor. Simple as it sounds, it plays an important role in the decision-making process as to how to best expedite your recovery. How people feel about their problem is important. They may understand it without even knowing the nature of their illness, but the fact that their problem is getting worse is important.

How well someone is sleeping is an indirect measure of the impact of the problem on their health status in general. And again, from a patient-centered standpoint, that is crucial on how you manage their situation.

Symptomatic treatment of these common problems, even when we do not know the cause, not only improves a person's quality of life, but it also helps address their fears, which could be very reassuring.

In the case of diarrhea, anti-diarrhea medications like Imodium, in my opinion, are not necessary because they hardly work and do not address the real issues, which are often loss of electrolytes and dehydration, which can be fatal if left untreated.

You can see why drinking fluids, especially preparations that contain electrolytes, such as Gatorade or Powerade, can help. Sodium and potassium are the electrolytes that are commonly lost through stools.

Taking probiotics to replenish the good flora in the bowel is also important. Sometimes diarrhea happens because of the overgrowth of the abdominal flora, and bringing in the good ones restores the balance.

But there are clues that may indicate that you are going downhill. When you feel dizzy, see blood in your stool, especially mixed in the stool, or when the diarrhea goes on for more than two weeks, it's time to see a health care professional if you have not yet done so.

Fever is another common symptom that people ask a lot of questions about. It is an indication of an invasion in the body, often of an infectious nature. The most dreaded complication of fever is febrile seizures in children. As the name implies, that is a seizure following high temperature. It is the main reason why doctors advise people to use a medication to bring down the fever. Anti-inflammatory and acetaminophen medications are commonly used to bring down fever.

However, two things indicate a juvenile fever is due to a serious illness: either the medication does not bring the fever down, or when the fever comes down to normal but the child still looks sick. The sick look is hard to explain. It's easily understood through experience. Most parents would say that their child has not been him- or herself or is just looking gloomy. A health care professional may find it difficult to figure out, because it depends on knowing how active the child had been to begin with. This is where parents, especially mothers, can even have an advantage over the health care professional. A good example is the child who is often very playful and suddenly just stops playing or looks listless and wears the gloomy look.

A fever that does not break after three days could also potentially be serious; it could be a bacterial rather than a viral illness. In such a situation, we would work to determine whether what initially seemed like a viral illness were instead a bacterial infection. Possibilities to consider, based on the case history and examinations, include ear infection, sinusitis, chest infection, meningitis, and many others.

Bacterial infections are often more serious than viral illnesses. In that case, many of the criteria of the downhill rule would be crucial. If the ten-year-old boy I discuss here looked sick and was not eating or drinking well; if the fever persisted despite medications like Tylenol or ibuprofen to bring down the fever for beyond three days of onset, the consequences could be serious. There may be additional symptoms, like headaches, chest pain, shortness of breath, abdominal pains, or others that cause worry and are clues that the boy is going downhill. Then it would be important to seek medical help, because if the problem is not dealt with appropriately, the result can be fatal.

I have also been asked by many people why a fever in a similar situation like the one presented here may go away and then come back. There could be something else to diagnose and treat, but quite often such recurrence is due to a superinfection. When the viral illness weakens the body and its immunity; often the lungs become prone to bacterial infection. Staphylococcus infection in the lungs is a possibility to look out for and treat in a timely fashion. But it could also be other kinds of bacterial infections in the upper respiratory tract, notably ear infections, sinusitis, meningitis, or others.

Treatments

1. Specific Treatment
- Bacterial Infection: antibiotics are effective because they can kill the bacteria.
- Viral Infection: antibiotics are ineffective because they cannot kill viruses.
2. Reducing Symptoms
- Specific treatment for the problem is the best option, but short of that, symptomatic relief makes us feel better and in some instances can prevent serious complications like febrile seizures in the case of fever in infants.
- Prevention of the spread of germs to others when an infection is suspected is crucial. Thus, hygiene is the mainstay here;

rigorous hand-washing or coughing into facial tissue and blowing your nose gently are important.

- Drink plenty of fluids too because it is important to stay hydrated. In case of diarrhea or vomiting, fluids with electrolytes are preferable.
- Try inhaling steam and using nasal spray decongestants and humidifiers.
- Take ibuprofen or acetylsalicylic acid (aspirin) or acetaminophen for pain.
- If you have allergies, avoid contact with things that can trigger an attack.

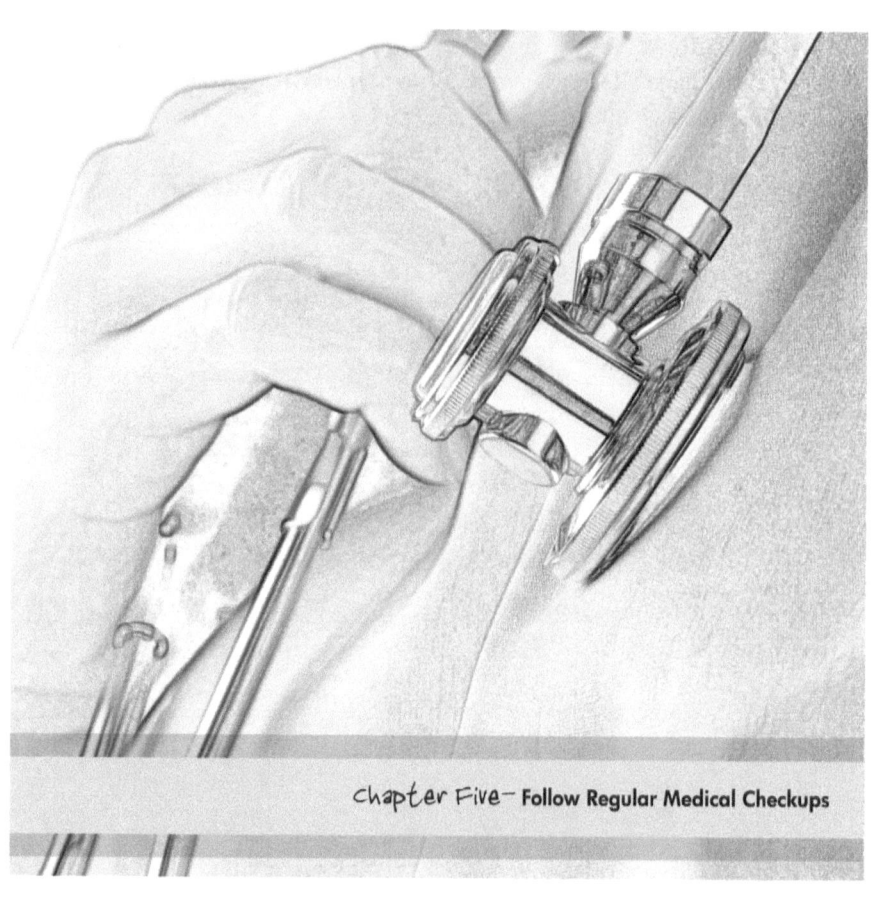

chapter Five— **Follow Regular Medical Checkups**

Chapter Five

Schedule Regular Medical Checkups

Lucky Harry never really cared about regular medical checkups until he had the heart attack scare, which got his attention. His wife told me that he came from the old-school frame of mind—don't fix it if it is not broken. I told him that I also believed in that, but it doesn't apply to seeing a health care professional for routine checkups. Besides, you have to evaluate whether it is broken before knowing when to fix it! As we spoke, the analogy of taking a car to the garage popped into my mind, and I asked him how often he took his car to the garage. Without missing a beat, he said twice each year.

Lucky Harry understood the analogy because it needed no additional clarification. I could see that Lucky Harry was attempting to be a model of restraint, and I did not want to continue preaching. His wife chimed in, saying that neglect and ignorance were more to the point.

She told me that *priority* was not in Lucky Harry's vocabulary. He would rather shampoo his dog than go see a doctor for a medical checkup.

There are too many Lucky Harrys in the world to count. Not too long ago, I saw a fellow in his fifties who was born and raised in North America. He told me that he had never had regular medical checkups. Luckily he had a motivator—his spouse who was concerned because he had been losing weight recently. To her knowledge, he was doing everything the same as he had been for a long time. There was no major change in his lifestyle.

And what was the lifestyle, you ask? He was a couch potato type. His blood pressure was through the roof. I wondered how this man had avoided a stroke. He was very lucky in that respect. But what I feared most was the severe weight loss. It turned out he had lung cancer that had metastasized to his neck with very big and ugly lumps. That was what his spouse was very worried about.

The rationale for regular medical checkups includes screening for early diagnosis and treatment of disease, if symptoms are not yet present. It is better to diagnose an ailment earlier than later, which tends to at least give people better quality of life or improve their chances of survival.

If this man had seen a doctor much earlier, like ten years before, his lung cancer would have been picked up much earlier too, and that could very well have saved his life. Ten years earlier, it might have been at its very initial stage and located in a small area of the lung that could have simply been removed surgically, possibly curing him.

When a cancer travels from the lungs to other parts of the body, like the neck and liver, then the person likely has a much shorter time to live. A poor prognosis for sure, but the reality. In this man's case, he had just a few months left to live.

Don't Forget the Follow-Ups

Following up after a diagnosis is another type of regular medical checkup. After Lucky Harry was diagnosed with a heart attack, he had to go for cardiac rehabilitation that involved a lot of different things. He needed to go to the doctor on a regular basis for his treatment optimization, including medication review, blood pressure check, graduated exercise on the treadmill to make sure that he does not put undue stress on his heart. Being proactive in this manner tends to be an important link in health care delivery because the patient has to be an instrument of positive influence. Why? Well, because his cooperation is needed. He is the one that often initiates the first step for getting care. Health care professionals are there to help people take care of their own health, but the people have to be the ones in the driver's seat.

Most of the things that are supposed to be done for regular medical checkups are tailored according to the age of the individual. Toward the end of this chapter, I will review the kinds of things that are relevant at each age, but if you do just one thing, contact a health care professional for a checkup! That is the most important thing; because they will educate you on what you should be doing. Keep in mind that recommendations may differ from professional to professional, as things in health care do change from time to time. Each person is unique. There may also be things that are peculiar to you.

Knowing the benefits of these checkups is also important. Many medical problems, like high blood pressure and diabetes, are often slow killers. Quite often the patient may not show any symptoms until it is too late. Various medical problems predispose people toward other health complications. For example, stress and high blood pressure usually go hand in hand. High blood pressure can cause stroke when it reaches a critical level. Slowly, over time, it damages other parts of your body, including your eyes, heart, kidneys.

I once found it difficult to convince a fellow in his fifties with high blood pressure to take medication and make a lifestyle change; he told me that he was feeling fine. But I explained to him that symptoms for high blood pressure may come at a later stage, when the organs have already been damaged. When his blood pressure was really through the roof, headaches and dizziness might occur.

A critical part of healthy living is to focus on long-term goals. But human nature lends itself to quick fixes and short-term pleasures. That is why being a model of restraint is crucial. You have to be able to subsume your urge for immediate gratification for long-term benefit.

So do not be like Lucky Harry, who said, "I feel good, so why see a doctor?" Well, he may not feel good a few years down the road. Do so on account of the potential benefits down the road. It is much less motivating when the gain is neither apparent nor immediate, but you'll know that it worked.

You can prevent future stroke or heart attack by acting today. Follow the instructions later in this chapter on how to master your emotions, use food as medicine rather than for gratification, and much more. If you see your health care professional, he or she could check you over, send you for screening tests and CRP (c-reactive protein).

If your cholesterol level is going up, for example, there are many things that can be done to correct it that will ward off future stroke or heart attack. Some people, like Lucky Harry, will wait until they have a stroke or a heart attack before seeing a doctor, at which time it might be too late, because the progressive deposition of cholesterol on the arteries in the heart and brain has blocked them. When the arteries are coated, their lumen size becomes narrower. When that reaches a critical level, it impedes blood flow into the different areas of the brain or heart. That is what leads to stroke, heart attack, or anginal pain. Sometimes a little piece of the material on the lining of the blood vessel called plaque breaks up and becomes lodged in the brain or heart, causing the same problem.

I lost a great patient to cancer of the colon. She had blood mixed in her stools, which was a tip off for possible bowel infection or cancer. Having a colonoscopy (scope) was necessary in order to screen for cancer. She refused to get the test done because she was too shy. She waited for a few years, during which time her family encouraged her to get it done. By the time she gained the courage to do the scope, it was too late. The cancer had spread from her colon to her liver and lungs. At the time of metastasis, the prognosis is guarded because, depending on the virulence of the cancer at that stage, the patient has only months to live, not years.

If she had been a little braver and went for the scope earlier, the cancer would have been recognized when it was still localized, before metastasis to a distant organ. Depending on the stage of discovery, a combination of surgery, chemotherapy, and/or radiation therapy could have solved the problem.

Quite often I tell my patients that a little bit of anxiety related to a medical checkup could be the price that they have to pay for saving their life. And if they visualize themselves enjoying the benefits of staying healthy, rather than worrying about what may be discovered, it will make them feel better about seeing their doctor.

Health care professionals are on the same team as their patients and share the same goal—keeping the patient healthy. So it is in each person's best interest to get checked. Knowing whether the patient has an ailment is better than being in the dark, especially if the ailment is one whose prognosis will get worse with time. It's hard for me to think of any medical problems that have a better prognosis the later it is discovered.

Often a quick stop to see a health care professional for a few questions and appropriate education can put a lot of fears to rest. And it is better to be reassured, rather than lie in bed and worry about an ailment that you may not even have. In such circumstances, I find that people tend to try and guess what their problem is. I know that such guesswork refuels doubt. These are all precursors to more stress and toxic (negative) emotions. These are joy-stealers!

The key to regular checkups is to see your doctor or health care professional to discover what is relevant for you. But there is nothing wrong in knowing a little more than the average person, so I will tell you the many kinds of tests that I recommend should be done according to a person's age.

Medical checkups and testing start at birth. It used to be thought that the time to stop regular testing was at seventy years old. But that is not generally true nowadays, because people tend to live much longer. So see your health care professional so you can find out when to stop routine screening. The way I look at it is that it should be tailored to your needs and how healthy you are.

For men fifty and older:
- Blood work, including cholesterol level, thyroid level, and blood sugar levels
- PSA (prostate specific antigen) for prostate cancer screening
- A colonoscopy every five years is recommended
- A rectal exam

Women fifty and older:
- Blood work, including blood sugar levels
- Thyroid level, cholesterol
- Ca-125 (ovarian cancer screening)
- Mammogram every two years
- Annual pap test

Women between eighteen and forty-nine:
- Blood work, including thyroid level
- Blood sugar level
- Cholesterol
- CRP (c-reactive protein)
- Annual pap tests
- If they have a first degree relative with breast or colon cancer, they will need a mammogram or colonoscopy, respectively, ten years earlier than the age that the family member was diagnosed.

Men between eighteen and forty-nine:
- Blood work, including thyroid level
- Blood sugar level
- CRP
- Cholesterol
- If there is a first degree relative with colon or prostate cancer,

they should start getting a colonoscopy and prostate screening, respectively, ten years before the age that the family member was diagnosed.

People below the age of eighteen are generally healthy, so they tend to see a health care professional only when needed. However, it is recommended that women under eighteen receive regular pap tests when they turn eighteen, or within two years after they start having sexual intercourse.

Birth control pills are commonly used to prevent pregnancy, regulate irregular menstruation cycles, or for very painful menses (cramps), when the use of an anti-inflammatory fails.

Birth control pills are about 99 percent effective. The common side effects are weight gain and headaches. It is often advised to use condoms in combination with the pill, which have an effectiveness of 90 percent. Condoms also protect against many sexually transmitted diseases. These include herpes simplex virus, gonococci, chlamydia, syphilis, and HIV.

Immunization to induce antibodies to strengthen the immunity in order to fight disease, notably infections, is very important. Some immunizations are licensed and some are not, so if you are not covered by a health insurance plan, there may be a cost to you for some of these vaccinations.

Immunization Schedule

Below is a detailed immunization schedule. Your health care professional can provide more information when necessary, but this list provides a guideline from which to build.

Immunization Schedule [12]

Two months old
- DTaP-IPV-Hib: diphtheria, tetanus, whooping cough, polio, hib
- Pneu-C-7: Pneumococcal disease

Four months old
- DTaP-IPV-Hib: Diphtheria, tetanus, whooping cough, polio, hib
- Pneu-C-7: Pneumococcal disease

---

12   Public Health Agency of Canada. 27 July 2010 <www.phac-aspc.gc.ca>

Six months old
- Influenza: The flu
- DTaP-IPV-Hib: Diphtheria, tetanus, whooping cough, polio, hib
- Pneu-C-7: Pneumococcal disease

Twelve months old
- Men-C: Meningococcal disease
- MMR: Measles, mumps, rubella

Fifteen months old
- Pneu-C-7: Pneumococcal disease
- Varicella: Chicken Pox

Eighteen months old
- DTaP-IPV-Hib: Diphtheria, tetanus, whooping cough, polio, hib
- MMR: Measles, mumps, rubella

Four to six years old
- DTaP-IPV: Diphtheria, tetanus, whooping cough, polio

Fourteen to sixteen years old
- DTaP-IPV: Diphtheria, tetanus, whooping cough, polio

Your primary care doctor will suggest the ones that are indicated in your situation; for example, you may need a hepatitis A and B vaccination if you are travelling to a developing country. Pneumococci vaccinations are offered to people who are predisposed to lung infections, as in those who have lost their spleen or people with chronic lung diseases or diabetes.

Influenza vaccinations and swine flu are most indicated in elderly people because of presumably low immunity levels. But the whole spectrum of indications often changes from year to year, for various reasons. It's important to stay current by contacting a health care professional.

It has been shown that immunizations have far more benefits than risks. A very minor part of the population tends to avoid them for controversial and personal reasons, notably fears of autism and Guillain-Barré syndrome. Some people believe that these conditions are caused by vaccinations.

The nature of the brain problems with autism is not known. Autism results in severe behavioral, intellectual, and communication problems. Experts say that autism happens to occur around the ages that the vaccinations are done, but no cause has been proven.[13] Hence it's appearance may just be a matter of timing. The same argument has been made for Guillain-Barré syndrome; it often presents around the same time as the flu vaccination and other viral illnesses. This disease causes ascending paralysis from the feet, legs, and lower abdomen. Paralysis means the loss of sensation, power, and tone in the muscles, which makes it difficult, if not impossible, to walk. It can also involve the upper spine, leading to paralysis of the respiratory muscles. Without prompt attention, like putting the patient on a ventilator to help him breathe, it can be fatal.

Recently a patient came to see me in my medical clinic because he was having severe headaches. They were heralded by a swine flu injection that he blamed for his ailment. After a complete case history and examination, we discovered that his blood pressure was severely elevated. The high blood pressure was likely the cause of his headaches. It took a lot to convince him that his high blood pressure was the reason for his ailment, not the vaccination he'd received. I bring up this point to illustrate that timing can be a very informative indicator of the cause of an illness, but we must keep in mind that sometimes it can just be a coincidence!

Regular checkups are another key step in staying healthy. In that respect, I like the saying "a stitch in time saves nine." If you ward off having colon cancer through early screening, you may save more than nine stitches. I know far too many people who have had cancer because they were too shy to go in for their regular medical checkup.

---

13   MMR vaccine. 26 July 2010. Wikipedia. 27 July 2010 < http:// en.wikipedia.org/wiki/MMR_vaccine>

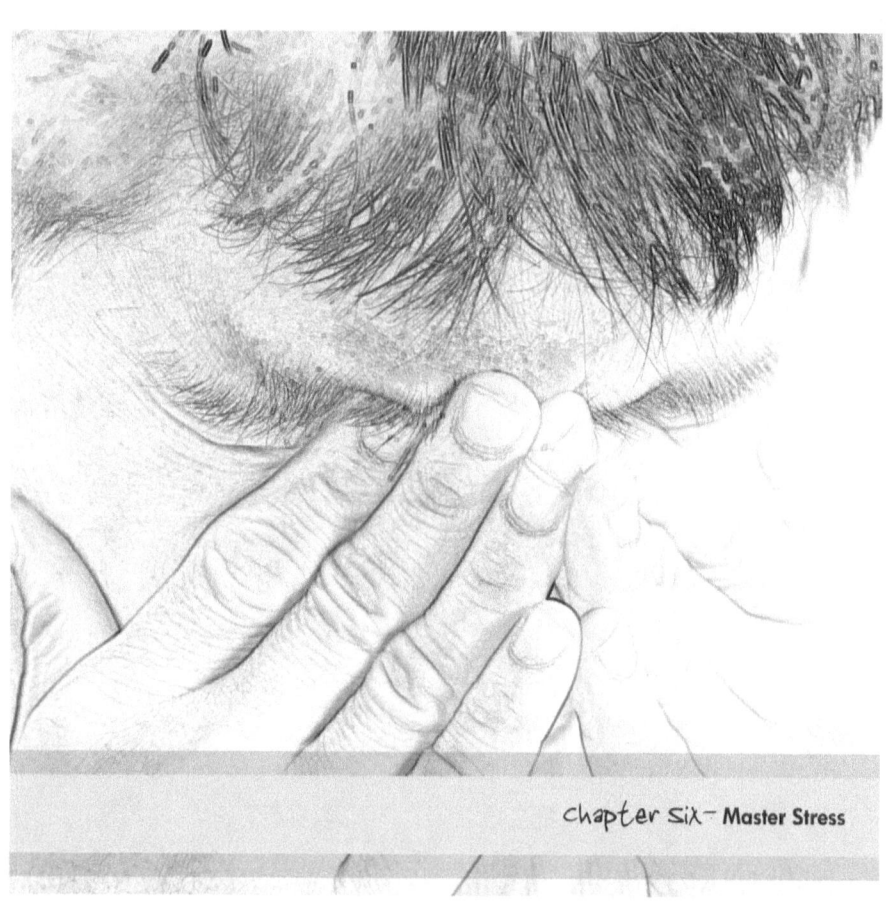

chapter six– **Master Stress**

Chapter Six

Master Stress

The Mechanism of Stress

William James, one of the early psychologists, demonstrated that the brain unconsciously monitors the body for changes and then interprets those changes according to what the situation seems to demand. James went on to suggest that all human emotions actually come from our perception of the physical condition that we are in—real or imagined. "We do not weep because we feel sorrow; we feel sorrow because we weep."[14]

So anxiety is the feeling of fear—imagined or real. Fear and anger are the expressions of tension and heightened involuntary autonomic nervous system response. The tension felt when afraid is a survival response. When you become frightened by a threat, there are two options: stay and fight or run away. Either way, the body needs to muster strength, with minimal voluntary control.

The fight or flight response is the body's instinctive survival reaction. The body goes into overdrive, to gain as much energy as possible. Physical energy comes from a chemical reaction between oxygen and blood sugars. Both of these are carried in the bloodstream to the muscles; effectively, the sugar is "burned" to produce energy. This process requires oxygen, so muscles in action need to have a continuous supply of fresh, oxygenated blood to work properly.

14   Seligman, Martin. *Authentic Happiness: Using the New Positive Psychology to Realize Your Potential for Lasting Fulfillment.* Free Press. 2003

As a result, many of the physical changes center around getting oxygen into the bloodstream. We breathe more deeply and more rapidly, increasing the oxygen supply entering the lungs. Blood pressure increases, carrying blood around the body much faster, and extra red blood cells, which carry oxygen, are released in to the bloodstream.

Some changes center on getting "fuel" to the muscles. Stored fats are converted into blood sugars and released into the bloodstream. The digestive system begins to work differently, ignoring long-term digestion and increasing the digestive process for rapidly acting foods such as sugars. Saliva in the mouth changes in the same way, so that we can metabolize rapid-energy foods quickly.

Another set of changes is designed to protect us from injury as much as possible. The amount of vitamin K in the blood increases, making the blood more able to clot quickly if there is an injury. Also, if we are very frightened, blood vessels close to the surface of the skin shrink, making us paler and minimizing the amount of blood we are likely to lose if we are injured. Blood supply to the vital internal organs of the body, on the other hand, increases.

We can see that the fight or flight response is a very powerful reaction that serves an important survival function when we are faced with threats that require physical response.

It is not quite as helpful when we are faced with non-physical threats, such as anxiety (fear of anticipated pain), like before seeing a dentist. Such threats do not require physical action, so we do not have a way of using up that energy and can quickly become stressed.

Arousal is a lesser degree of the fight or flight response. When our attention is caught by something or when we feel anxious about something, we experience the same kinds of physical changes but to a much lesser degree.

Arousal means that a lot of physical responses are stimulated simultaneously. The type of arousal we experience with fear is slightly different from the type we experience when we are angry, but the two conditions have a great deal in common.

Fight or flight response is an extreme state of physiological arousal. But there are less extreme forms of arousal as well. Arousal thus exists in terms of a continuous scale, which has extreme relaxation at one end, and fight or flight at the other. Many arousal levels fall in between. A disagreement or any worrying thought can make us more aroused.

Arousal is not necessarily a bad thing, because a small amount of arousal is stimulating; up to a point, increased arousal helps us perform better. For example, a bit of irritation during an argument can help us find words easily and talk more eloquently. Many people consume a beverage with caffeine or do exercise because the additional stimulation helps them feel more alert.

If we become too aroused—perhaps becoming very angry or, worse, enraged by a situation—it can impair our performance in a situation. There are distinct physiological differences between the kind of arousal produced by fear and anger and that produced by feeling uplifted (joy). These differences seemed to be the result of different hormones and brain chemicals involved in the different emotions.[15] Both fear and anger involve a chemical named adrenaline, but anger also involves another one, known as noradrenalin.

Adrenaline and noradrenalin are both chemicals used by the body to stimulate a special part of the nervous system, known as the autonomic nervous system. This consists of a network of nerve fibers running to all the internal organs of the body. When the part of the autonomic nervous system known as the sympathetic division is stimulated, the body experiences arousal. However, when the other part, known as the parasympathetic division, is stimulated, the body becomes quieter and less active. The parasympathetic division seems to be involved in quiet emotions such as depression.

Stimulating the vagis nerve, a major pathway between the body and the brain, causes the release of oxytonin, a feel-good hormone.

Stress

If we become angry with someone or experience a fight response, the emotion often passes. We calm down and get over it. As we do so, the physical symptoms of arousal disappear as well. But sometimes we can experience emotional arousal that doesn't go away. Being anxious about whether there will be enough money to pay the bills, for instance, is a continuous worry, not a passing thing. This means that it's constantly producing physiological arousal that doesn't go away. Long-term arousal

---

15   Amen, Daniel G. *Making a Good Brain Great: The Amen Clinic Program for Achieving and Sustaining Optimal Mental Performance.* Three Rivers Press. 2006.

such as this can have harmful effects, including interfering with both our psychological and physical health. We call it stress.

Long-term stress suppresses the body's immune system, making us much more vulnerable to illness. Long-term stress also makes us nervous. It makes us fear potential threats. This attitude of being on the edge means that we may see something as a threat when it is really quite harmless.

This state of mind also makes us overact to what people do. In that way we become more likely to quarrel with people around us. It also affects our judgment, as our decisions are more likely to be less sensible. We can use coping mechanisms to minimize the effects of long-term stress, as we learn to deal with problems in a positive way.

Stress can feed into the fight-flight response, which is actually an instantaneous defense mechanism for the whole body. The stimulus from stress makes us more alert, in anticipation of danger, if there is real danger. So increased arousal from stress, up to a point, helps us to do things better—moderate quantities of adrenaline are very important for priming and getting you ready for action.

The sources of environmental stress, like crowding, noise, and traffic jams, are numerous. Any form of disaster or accidents fall on this category of massive stress.

Another category of events is called *stressors*. These are things that happen to us that are likely to increase our level of stress. These include anything from loss of a job, loss of a loved one, diagnosis of a serious disease, separation from a loved one, and poor cash flow, to name a few. These losses can be either real or imagined.

Irrespective of the factors that cause stress, stress affects your level of arousal, so that you feel on edge and often irritable rather than released. A lot of studies done by psychologists, notably by Glass and Singer in 1972, show that if we feel that we have some control over the stimuli around us, then we don't find them nearly as stressful. So, a sense of control is the key in reducing stress.

If fear is a feeling that we choose, choose confidence instead. Facing a situation with confidence makes your brain release pleasure chemicals, like dopamine and serotonin, that will boost your level of enthusiasm and banish your fears.

In your attempt to make lifestyle changes, take one step at a time.

If you run your whole day's work or life like a movie in front of you, it becomes very overwhelming. You may tackle daily exercise to relieve stress. You could take another small step by eating a balanced diet, reducing your caffeine intake, or avoiding recreational drugs, which tend to make stress worse through withdrawal from the substances. It has been my experience that some people make too many changes at a time, and that overwhelms them. When you eat an apple, you take one bite at a time and don't put the whole apple into your mouth!

Locus of Control

We can use coping mechanisms to minimize the effects of long-term stress, as we learn to deal with problems in a positive way. The essence of a coping strategy is to control the amount of arousal that you experience, either physical or psychological, as they involve thinking in some way. These may include mental exercises and ways of using your imagination positively. Thoughts that feel bad create negative emotions like guilt, envy, jealousy, which simply add to the amount of stress which you feel.[16]

Visualization is very important in stress management. By concentrating on positive thoughts and imagining yourself happy, you leave no mental room for anxiety. If you want to be healed from an ailment, imagine yourself without the ailment. If you want to use this method to make your life much less stressful, see yourself without the stressor. Visualize the happy ending.[17]

People often add to the stress they feel by thinking negatively. They may worry about how dreadful things may become, because anxiety is the feeling of fearing or anticipating something bad. All thinking of this kind adds to our level of arousal and stress. Negative thoughts lead to negative emotions, which draw pain or suffering toward you in the form of psychological resistance. Psychological resistance eclipses the flow of well-being.

Whenever you feel negative emotions, stop and change the thought to one that feels good. This is how you make yourself happy, by focusing on the things that feel good or energize you. Good-feeling thoughts put you in harmony with your broader perspective—your soul, or who you really are.

---

16   Nkut, Dr. Alfred. *Leadership for Success: A Dynamic Model of Influence.* AuthorHouse. 2010.
17   Amen, Daniel G. *Making a Good Brain Great: The Amen Clinic Program for Achieving and Sustaining Optimal Mental Performance.* Three Rivers Press. 2006.

So, the best way to break the vicious cycle of negativism is to reach for a good-feeling thought. You will experience relief from the tension and an improved emotional response.

Attributions are the reasons that we give for why things happen. Someone with a depressive attributional style will believe anything that happens will only turn out for the worse. Those negative thoughts keep their depression going, partly because it makes them feel helpless and hopeless. This frame of mind makes them feel more anxious because they believe that they are not in control of what happens in their lives. People with a depressive attributional style have an external locus of control. They believe that they cannot influence what happens to them.

People with different attributional styles, who see themselves as able to control events, either through their thoughts or efforts, don't easily give up. They experience stress differently. They take active control over their lives because they know that they are the instrument of their own destiny. They are much less likely to become depressed and much more likely to do something about their situation. These people have what is known as an internal locus of control. They believe that what happens to them is their own responsibility.

Having an internal locus of control is much healthier for a human being—both physically and mentally. Long-term stress can lower the body's resistance to disease and make us vulnerable to illness. People with an internal locus of control experience much less stress. This is because they channel their energies into looking for positive things to do instead of just worrying, and because they are likely to gain at least a measure of success through trying so hard, they experience positive emotions, such as a sense of achievement, that people who are more passive don't feel.

More joy comes from performing a service that you feel positive about than the service per se. Your positive perceptions cause your brain to release chemicals that make you happier, like dopamine and serotonin. Incremental achievements or successes make you feel uplifted, and this shifts your emotional set-point upward— you feel happier.

Those who believe they have an external locus of control allow external factors or circumstances to have undue influence on them. For example, two people may be faced with a stressful life event, like bereavement. The person who reacts to the situation will attract more psychological suffering. The person who exercises more control, constantly affirming his confidence and high self-esteem, is rewarded when his brain releases pleasure chemicals that further boost his level of happiness. He is more stable than the former person. The former person reacts to the bereavement, and that can easily lead to depression. Why? Because depression is the feeling of loss often triggered by lack of confidence and low self-esteem. That is what often leads to the feeling of inadequacy in depression. Remember that happiness is the image within that we create and project to our outer world. What we believe and affirm is what we become.

Quite often you need at least twenty-one days to get a habit installed. Another way is through a strong emotional occurrence that moves you out of your comfort zone. To wait for that is to live by default, rather than by design. If a mishap shakes you up and becomes a wake-up call for you, that's fine. But you can learn from other people's experiences and move forward by installing habits that you deem important to your quest for happiness.

Cognitive therapy is all about teaching people how to take control of their lives. It also teaches them how to avoid the self-defeating beliefs and attributions that have stopped them from doing so in the past. Almost anything that increases someone's self-esteem has the effect of giving them more of an internal locus of control over their own life, helping them to cope with stressful problems positively. Problems may be real and not likely to go away, but we can make their effects on us worse or better, depending on how we deal with them. This is why attitude is more powerful than facts.

We have more positive emotions than we sometimes realize, and those may be associated with small as well as big events. Awareness of the different types of positive emotions we can create is important; knowing these different types of positive emotions will make you better at navigating your emotions. Awareness often precedes action. Staying above the fray is the key to happiness. A lot of unhappiness comes from trying to resist situations. It often draws psychological pain or resistance to you. It is very easy to create any of these emotions because the context is very obvious.

Simply reach for positive-feeling thoughts that simulate these situations when you are preoccupied or obsessed by those states of mind; it basically crowds out the negative emotions. Make affirmations, visualize yourself the way you want to be, and practice over and over in order to make it your dominant feeling.

The first emotion is simply feeling a sense of confidence—feeling capable and able to do whatever is needed. The key is to focus on what you can do, not on what you cannot do through a sense of spirituality or wonder. It might be anything that resonates with your inner being, like God being the provider of abundance in all areas of your life. It could be something as simple as enjoying nature or a great piece of art work.

Feel contentment or relaxation as well, as opposed to being tense. Researchers have reported self-indulgence could just be a simple pleasure for you—a treat for yourself. Altruism is another positive emotion that is related to sharing or caring for other people.

Being interested in something or fascinated by a hobby is also a type of emotion that people enjoy experiencing, referred to as *absorption*. Exhilaration is also described, the sort of emotion one would feel when excited about something or thrilled by an unexpected pleasant experience.

Stress-Related Diseases

When I first met Lucky Harry, he was very knowledgeable, yet he had his blind spots. He talked about his boss being a major source of stress in his life because he was a control freak who was nagging all the time. Until I had the opportunity to actually speak with him to assess how much of a stressor his boss' behavior was to him, I did not know. I found out that Lucky Harry was right. His concern was real; it was not mere imagination or exaggeration on his part.

What Lucky Harry did not understand was the fact that stress is a major risk factor for his medical problems: heart attack, diabetes, and obesity. I am not trying to say that stress contributed 100 percent, but understanding the physiology of how stress contributes to the major killers in our world will make more sense.

Research shows that about 50 percent of the weight that we carry is genetically determined (the genetic set-point theory.[18]) However, the other 50 percent, which is environmentally related, can, to some degree, be handled by us, and that is what is important. How we make choices on a daily basis is the power of control that we do have. And that is the part that is crucial, because we can change it!

When Lucky Harry learned the connection between stress and his medical problems, he became more enthusiastic about doing something about it. I think that people are going to be more motivated to act when they understand why they are doing what they are doing. And even more

18   Set Point Theory. Centre for Clinical Interventions. 27 July 2010 < www. cci.health.wa.gov.au>

importantly, when they see the benefits upfront, it further motivates them. I feel that knowledge, unless it serves the purpose of giving us a kick on the chin to act, it's just a myth! Only action eventually moves us forward; knowledge does not, on its own.

A stressor is anything or situation that causes you stress. It could be of any nature: social, psychological, emotional, physical, or medical. For example, a diagnosis of cancer or loss of a job constitutes major stressors. Lucky Harry's nagging boss was a major source of stress.

But what is stress? *Stress* is the term for your body's reaction to feelings of pressure. Stress in our hectic lives is a reality that we must understand, along with how it affects our bodies. Otherwise we will not know how to deal with it.

Stress could be caused by both good and bad circumstances, like being called for a good job or having a nagging boss, respectively. Stress from a good situation can motivate and energize you. But negative or prolonged stress can be bad for your health.

The things that don't bother you at all could be very stressful for someone else. Therefore, our perception of the stressor determines whether the event is a source of motivation or not. It also determines the size of our fight or flight response, the psychological response to danger that is either perceived or real. You can see why some people when confronted with a rattlesnake stimulate this mechanism to the point that the fear may even make them faint! But other people minimize this response with a positive attitude toward the snake.

Note that part of the phobia related to the rattlesnake may be unconscious. That is, the long-term memory in the subconscious mind may be responding subliminally to the messages that you have implanted there in the past about not liking rattlesnakes. But either way, what you tell yourself about the stressor (using autosuggestion) is important.

Autosuggestion is also defined as unconsciously influencing your behavior. This is why speaking to ourselves shortly before falling asleep is a very powerful to influence on our internal dialogue. Saturating our conscious mind with what we want wills it to the subconscious, which is the seat of our long-term memory and is associated with habit forming. Unless the adult who is afraid of rattlesnakes reconditions himself by repeated positive affirmations for a long time, he will continue to react unconsciously to the snakes in a negative way.

So again, our perception and degree of apprehension to the stressor will determine the scale of the fight or flight response. This is a primitive physiological response that was meant for self-preservation and protection. So in the face of clear danger, whether real or imagined, the brain triggers this response.

Adrenaline increases our heart rate and breathing in order to increase oxygen to the body, while the cortisol stimulates the release of glucose, fat, and amino acids into the bloodstream for energy production. But that is not the problem. The issue is excessive or long-term exposure of the body to high levels of these stress hormones.

So any chronic source of stress can keep these hormones at levels too high for you to keep up with. It is a vicious cycle, because high cortisol increases your stress level, and high stress also increases your cortisol level. But chronic stress is very complicated; it decreases very complex biochemical pathways and testosterone and growth hormone levels. This causes the body to store fat, lose muscle, slow down metabolism, and increase appetite. You can see how stress is working against your effort to be fit or manage your weight!

In a stressful situation, real or imagined, the pituitary gland stimulates the adrenal gland to release adrenaline and cortisol. Long-term exposure to high levels of cortisol are unequivocally associated with elevated cholesterol levels, heart disease, hypertension, lowered libido, poor concentration, diabetes (reduced sensitivity to insulin), and it decreases immune system function by suppressing lymphocyte activity(a type of white blood cell that secretes immunoglobulin) to fight disease in the body.

The effects of stress are innumerable, but we can understand why the presence of excessive stress in our lives triggers depression, anxiety, tension headaches, and tension in the muscles, especially in the shoulders and neck area.

Also, when facing these stressful events, the emotional center of your brain, the limbic system, is stimulated and leads to negative emotions, like fear, anger, frustration, and depression.

And what about tension or aches in the muscles? When facing a stressful event, the premotor area in the brain is stimulated. This area of the brain controls movement of the muscles. Impulses in the brain will tell the muscles to get ready for action. That is why they tighten up in response to the stressor. This exaggerated effect leads to tensing and pain in the muscles when we feel stressed out.[19]

---

19   Thomas E. Andreoli, Charles C. J. Carpenter, Robert C. Griggs, Joseph Loscalzo. *Cecil Essentials of Medicine*. Saunders, 2003.

What Determines Stress?

I believe that in order to adequately deal with stress, we have to know the things that create stress and be able to figure out whether we have the symptoms, what to do about it, and then do it!

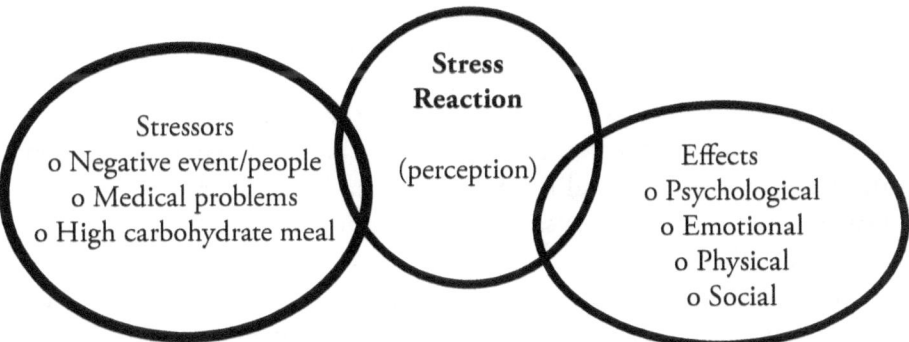

Stress Reaction

Stressors
o Negative event/people
o Medical problems
o High carbohydrate meal

(perception)

Effects
o Psychological
o Emotional
o Physical
o Social

How to Determine Stress

I have already explained how these factors feed into the vicious cycle of the stress hormone response, leading to chronic stress. I would like to emphasize why a high carbohydrate meal is a physiological stressor.

In times of stress, your body breaks down fat, carbohydrates, and protein to create energy in response to whatever is troubling you. You will experience a rise in glucose, free fatty acids, and cholesterol. Because of the increased glucose circulating in your blood, the pancreas will secrete insulin to counteract it. The insulin will break down the sugar in the blood, leading to low blood sugar levels. This could lead to feelings of hunger, fatigue, and irritability.

Low blood sugar is a physiological stressor that stimulates your body to secrete even more cortisol, raising the blood sugar again, hence repeating the vicious cycle. In the body, carbohydrates are broken down before the fat and proteins by the stress hormones. Here is the most interesting part.

What you eat matters, so strive for a balance between carbohydrates and proteins in your diet. This is very easy. Aim for putting proteins and carbohydrates on your plate in the ratio of about 1:1—equal portions of each. Because carbohydrates are physiologic stressors, they make your body secrete insulin and store fat. That makes you crave more sugars or carbohydrates to make sure that you have enough energy to defend yourself.

That is why carbohydrates are generally for fuel. They are processed and stored when taken in excess.

On the other hand, proteins make your body secrete glucagon, a hormone that modulates the effect of insulin and makes your body burn more fat. So the proteins together with carbohydrates reduce the intensity of those carbohydrates as a physiological stressor.

You can see how you can lose more weight with better food choices. Note that vegetables and fruits are considered carbohydrates too.

That is part of what I mean when I say that you should view food as medicine. Indeed, what you eat affects your chemistry—in this situation, the stress hormones insulin and glucagon. These hormones are very instrumental in disease causation and weight control. This is explained in the next chapter.

And where your calories come from matters. One of the biggest myths is that where your calories come from does not matter. Wrong. It does matter, as I have already shown you. The vicious cycle of stress hormones leading to the sugar blues—fatigue and poor concentration that comes from a dip in your sugar levels following a release of insulin that breaks down the sugars in your blood—is made worse when you eat carbohydrates with high glycemic index. Why? Because when carbohydrates have a high glycemic index, the sugar from them goes into your bloodstream very fast. Refined sugar (table sugar) and glucose, for example, help accelerate this cascade.

So you are advised to eat mainly complex carbohydrates with a low glycemic index, which is very important. So yes, your food choices can affect your stress level.

Stress is infectious and can affect almost any aspect of your life, even in very subtle ways. It is a slow killer. It affects our blood pressure in an insidious manner; eventually hypertension, a primary factor in stroke causation, can put you in a wheelchair if it causes a stroke.

Quite often, people say to me that they feel good, and they do not think that they need to do anything for their blood pressure. But sometimes people come into my clinic because they are bleeding from the nose or have excruciating headaches or slurred speech, which means there is a good chance that they are having or about to have a stroke or mini-stroke.

Stress is such a great imitator that you may not even realize that it is what is killing you very slowly, either through disease causation or by slowly eating away at your personal relationships through the change in your emotions, like anger and frustration, that infect everything you do.

Stress can even affect your internal dialogue because it is also associated with negative thinking.

Excess stress can also lead to extreme feelings of sadness, change in sleep patterns, poor decision making, insomnia, and changes in weight and appetite.

Tips for Coping with Stress

Tip #1: Normalization

When you find yourself in a stressful situation, the first thing to do is to normalize it—say to yourself that stress is a normal part of life. This positive self-talk will help your body not react so extremely to the stressor and minimize your fight or flight response. Remember that whether your intention is to fight or run, this alert system puts the body in overdrive in order to protect itself. It is a self-preservation mechanism. That is when the stress hormones, notably adrenaline and cortisol, are secreted by the adrenal glands.

You can see how perception changes your chemistry. So how you perceive the event is key to the degree of the body's response. Seeing it as a threat makes it a stressor!

The placebo effect (as discussed in Chapter Three) shows that perception strongly affects our chemistry. A placebo is a substance with no medical properties; it has no physical positive or negative effect on the body. It has been shown that the using placebo effect in the treatment of any ailment works about 30 percent of the time. What this means is that if you diagnose a certain number of people with pain and give half of them a placebo for treatment (without their knowledge of it being a placebo rather than medication), about three out of ten of those people will tell you that they feel less pain. Testing has shown that those people on the placebo who actually believed it would work for the pain secreted high levels of endorphins, which has similar pain relief properties to morphine.

So, the verdict is that our perception strongly affects our chemistry. It affects the happy chemicals like serotonin, oxytocin, and dopamine as well as the fight or flight chemicals.

Tip #2: Autosuggestion

This is what we tell ourselves all day long. It determines our internal dialogue. Remember the story of the man and the rattlesnake? Those who get extreme responses from the body do so because they have internalized a danger. The extreme reaction may seem irrational to our reasoning mind, but it is important to know that the person may not even be aware of what is happening, because it is happening unconsciously. The subconscious mind has taken control.

Belief is very strong! The man near the rattlesnake has already internalized his response in the seat of his long-term memory. And unless he reconditions himself by using his reasoning mind with positive affirmations over time, he will not rise above his fear of snakes. So he needs reprogramming of the mind.

Tip #3: Teach Yourself to Relax

Focus on your muscles and whole body. But start with your mind. Detoxify your mind by focusing on the positive aspects of your life. That disarms the premotor area so that it does not send messages to your muscles to tense up. Your mind works by the power of affirmation, so it can only say yes to what you tell it, whether it be positive or negative. So crowd out the negative aspects of your life by focusing on the bright side. That is how you detoxify your life: by removing negative thinking and emotions that sap your energy. Instead, focus on the positive images and the things that you want in life. A lot of despair comes from perceived failures, past and the future.

Actions, like smiling, also help relieve tension. By tensing and relaxing your muscles, you can also relieve the strain in them. Remember that whatever you do through your imagination or actions to induce a relaxation state is synonymous with happiness— you are happy when you are relaxed! When you are tense, you're obviously not happy. Another simple way of relaxing and releasing tension from the muscles is to make a habit of breathing deeply all the time.

Tip #4: Exercise

Exercise is a great stress reliever. It is not necessary to wait until you are feeling stressed out before you do it. You can actually stay ahead of the game by exercising in order to ward off being stressed-out.

My experience has been that those who say that they do not have time to exercise are often the ones that crash later. They do not take time to build the strength that the body needs, so when the storm of a crisis comes, they are unprepared.

Integrating exercise with your lifestyle makes you look fit, manages your weight, and improves your longevity too. Those are additional benefits to getting out there and just doing it. Exercise is a positive distraction from worry as well as stress. It increases your energy and enthusiasm.

Visualize the psycho-spiritual benefits of exercise in order to get yourself into motion.

I do not care what kind of exercise you do because I am more interested in getting you out there. However, aerobic exercises will help you burn calories and also build cardio-respiratory endurance.

When you feel stressed out, get out and commune with nature—simply exercise. Go walking or biking, hike in the woods, or do whatever activity seems fun for you. I think that daily activity for about one hour per day, tempered by your specific needs, is good.

Setting the bar high fires you up. But you have to be realistic—even a fifteen-minute walk each day is better than nothing.

Tip #5: Rest

Lack of rest leads to high cortisol levels in your body consistent with high stress. If it goes on for a long period of time, it can lead to the stress-related diseases discussed earlier. Do whatever you need to do in order to get rest—sleep, take a holiday, or take a stress leave from work.

In some cases, it may be a good idea to consider taking over-the-counter sleep aids or prescription drugs that will help you sleep. Inadequate sleep or rest can lead to burnout and even depression. So the use of sleeping pills is sometimes advisable. Some over-the-counter sleep aids, such as melatonin, are natural hormones without potential side effects. But generally speaking, it's good to speak to your health care provider about lack of sleep because there could be secondary causes to screen for and treat.

Tip #6: Spirituality

This has to do with building inner strength. It is important to be recharged before you run out of steam. Quite often, burnout happens because we neglect building our strength; then we collapse under the least stressor.

You do not have to do anything in particular to be spiritual. Anything can be a spiritual practice, depending on your creed and attitude.

The key to spirituality is to bring yourself into harmony with the universe so that blessings unfold naturally. How? By focusing on a spiritual practice, we tune out the "noise" that often clouds our judgment, putting us into more direct access with our natural well-being.

Meditation, yoga, prayer, visualization, or any other spiritual practice of your choice will help you focus on positive emotions of peace and calm, instead of tension.

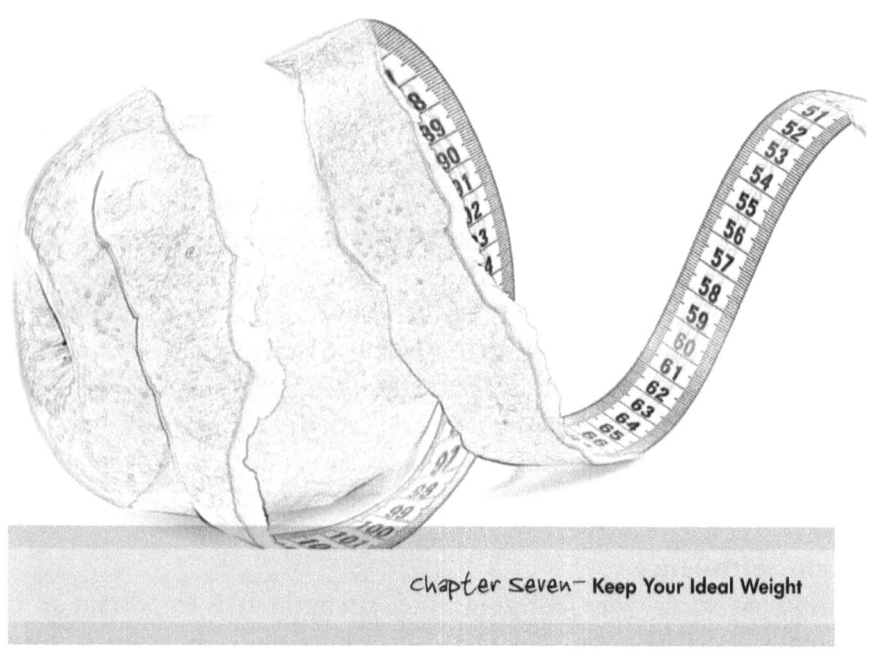

chapter seven— **Keep Your Ideal Weight**

Chapter Seven

Keep Your Ideal Weight

Lucky Harry was not a model of restraint. His wife confided in me that he had given up the fight to maintain an ideal weight. Part of the problem was the limiting beliefs and myths that he held.

He inherited his apple-shaped body from his parents for sure, but I kept reminding him that the genetic set-point for weight and shape of the body only accounted for 50 percent of the problem. He also thought that he was too fat to exercise.

But the biggest problem of all was his belief in the myth that as long as the food he ate was low fat, it will not make him gain weight. With such a false belief, he made no effort to control the portion sizes of his meals, which is the crux of weight control—the balance between the calories that he took in and those that he burned.

Lucky Harry was full of excuses and limiting ideas that held him back. So the best approach for him was to first debunk some of the myths by educating himself on the facts and avoiding the hype about weight management. Then came the process of helping him match his behavior with the goals he set in order to achieve it. And finally I provided practical tips for him to rise to the challenge. He used affirmations extensively in order to recondition as well as pace his life.

It is no joke that obesity is the number one public health problem in North America today. Within the past decade, the prevalence across all ages has doubled. It went from about 12 percent to 25 percent from about the year 2000 to 2010.[20] Consider that about 50 percent of the people that you know are overweight, and they have trouble controlling their weight. Lucky Harry is not alone, as you can see.

Generally speaking, obesity is defined as being more than 20 percent above your ideal weight. Later on in this chapter, I will give you more information on how to figure out your ideal weight.

But remember that we are genetically programmed for a set body shape and weight. That accounts for about 50 percent of what determines your weight. The rest of the factors are environmental. Our focus is to handle what we can control—the environmental factors. That is where self-motivation comes into the equation. Because we have to be willing to make the move and turn theory into action.

During my sessions with Lucky Harry, the most frequently asked question was how to control appetite. He told me that he was hungry all the time. He could not stop thinking about food.

Besides giving him the short answer—the affirmation "I feel satisfied," to repeat to himself all day long and shortly before falling asleep at night—I realized that it would make more sense if I educated him to understand the physiology of hunger.

Appetite control is a very complex process. Review Chapter Six for information on how hormones affect appetite. The satisfaction and hunger mechanism is controlled by the command center of the body in the brain—the hypothalamus. The hypothalamus controls many biological functions in your body, including your metabolism, appetite, temperature, sex drive, sleep, thirst, and much more. The satiety center in the hypothalamus regulates your appetite. It is influenced by the leptin and ghrelin hormones. The two hormones work in concert. Leptin acts as the hormone of satisfaction in shutting down appetite, and ghrelin does the opposite.

The balance between the two opposing impulses determines whether you feel hungry or not. Lucky Harry's big appetite was driving him crazy, so his anger became a stressor that refuelled the cortisol mechanism described in Chapter Six. Adrenaline and cortisol are stress hormones. They are put into our bloodstream by the adrenal glands that are regulated by the hypothalamus in the brain. Our perception affects our chemistry, so negative emotions like anger trigger the secretion of these stress hormones,

---

20   Obesity and overweight. World Health Organization. 27 July 2010 < http://www.who.int/dietphysicalactivity/publications/facts/obesity/en/>

which significantly increase the chance of developing major cases of death like obesity, diabetes (low insulin sensitivity), hearth attacks, high blood pressure, and stroke. So you can see why poor Lucky Harry could not win! The ghrelin hormone was winning.

The command center in the brain is v instrumental in ideal weight control, via its regulation of the satisfaction and hunger mechanisms. I told Lucky Harry that since his biology and his physiology did not favor him, he had to use psychology. Learning how to become a model of restraint was important. But as you can see, it was not as simple as putting a padlock on his mouth.

Another hot issue for Lucky Harry was that his appetite control was getting worse with age. I felt badly for him, because he had to learn the science behind his proclivity to gain more weight with age. It has been shown that as people get older, they have fewer leptin receptors in the hypothalamus. This correlates with fewer satiety signals, which makes these people prone to gaining more weight.[21]

Keeping aware is important in making a difference, because the only purpose that information serves us is to move us to action. In order to use information to that end, we must see the connection between it and how it benefits us.

Lucky Harry learned that he had to start looking at food and exercise as medications, because they actually affect our body in the same way that medications do. Their optimal use gives us longevity, reduces our risk for common killer diseases, and much more. The benefits of maintaining an ideal weight by eating modestly and exercising cannot be overemphasized.

Exercise not only reduces risks for depression, it also helps those who have depression recover. Exercise increases the survival rate for heart attack victims, relieves stress, and boosts enthusiasm and energy.

You have now learned how food triggers the satisfaction and hunger mechanisms and the physiology of weight control. So treat food as medication! How is this useful? The point here is that you should direct your thoughts and images to long-term satisfaction, not instant gratification. You should subject the urge to having dessert and sweets to your willpower. A good affirmation is to say to yourself that the dessert tastes good but makes you prone to a disease like diabetes later.

You can also decide to eat until simply you feel satisfied, not overly

---

21   Oz, Dr. Mehmet, Michael Dr. Roizen. *You: On A Diet: The Insider's Guide to Easy And Permanent Weight Loss.* Thorsons/Element. 2010

full. Constantly repeat to yourself, "I feel satisfied." Remember the role of autosuggestion in reconditioning your habits. Mindfulness about food being medication is important because we do not take medication for comfort. So do not eat for comfort either. That is why counting calories keeps you aware of how much you are putting in your mouth. You can always tell yourself that the extra calories on your plate are better off in the garbage can than around your belly.

One of the tips for preventing the common killer diseases is to live as if you have them already. In general, healthy eating habits and daily exercise will significantly reduce your risk for developing these diseases. But before embarking on a healthy eating and exercise plan, first assess your needs by doing the clinical assessment described in Chapter Two. The assessment will tell you the appropriate dieting regimen to follow. If you can understand Lucky Harry's clinical profiling, yours will be very easy, because his is a very complex case. However, the balanced diet regimen is the default regimen for those who are generally fit and want to continue to stay fit.

If you are in doubt of what to do, contact a health care professional to help assess your needs and provide support and motivation that you need to succeed.

It is common knowledge heart disease is the number one case of death in North America.[22] [23] And being obese more than doubles your chances. Being overweight also increases your risk for other common killer diseases, such as diabetes, stroke, anxiety, and cancer.

The benefits of keeping an ideal weight are astronomical. It also improves your sex life. How? Weight control improves the level of the sex hormone testosterone in your body. When fat is burned, it reduces the amount of testosterone converted into the female hormone, estrogen. This happens in both men and women because they both have testosterone. The main difference is that men have more of it than women. In the same way, women have more estrogen than men. This is why we generally look at testosterone as the male hormone and estrogen as the female hormone.

Healthy eating and exercise also reduces your cholesterol and blood sugar levels and increases your serotonin levels, the hormone that makes you happy.

---

22   Heart Disease. 15 April 2010. Centres for Disease Control and Prevention. 27 July 2010 <www.cdc.gov/nchs/fastats/heart.htm>

23   Leading Cause of Death and Hospitalization in Canada. Public Health Agency of Canada. 27 July 2010 <www.phac-aspc.gc.ca/publicat/lcd-pcd97/table1-eng.php>

Tips for Maintaining an Ideal Weight

Tip #1: Clinical Profiling and Assessment

First, figure out your dietary needs. See Chapter Two for more details about doing your own clinical assessment using Lucky Harry's case as an example. It involves simply deciding what diet regiment to go on.

Tip #2: Set a Clear Goal

If you want to be among the half of North Americans who have a handle on their weight, the key is to set a long-term goal. It sounds simple, but it is the cornerstone of building a successful healthy lifestyle. Long-term goals get you to your destiny. Why? Because goals are the fire lighters! They help program as well as pace your life for you.

Consider a soccer game without any goal posts. Imagine a game where all the twenty-two players run around aimlessly on the field because they have no goal (no net) to work toward. Think of the excitement that everybody gets when a goal is scored. That excitement does not exist without the goal.

But another very important key in succeeding is knowing the power of small steps. It is the small actions steps on a daily basis that carry you to the top. It is my "small bang theory" of leadership. Unfortunately there are people who believe in achieving things through one giant step. No. It is a recipe for failure. It is a way of programming yourself to fail.

If you want to program yourself for success, adopt the small bang theory. Each day take a positive step in the right direction. It does not matter how small the action step is; the point is that with time small steps have a compounding effect. They are also the recipe for overcoming the destructive negative habit of procrastination.

Also, once an action is begun, it leads to more self-motivation. For example, when you passi on dessert at dinner today, it is a small step that inspires subsequent action, and it is doing these small actions on a daily basis that eventually gives you the trim figure that you are seeking. Each time you are tempted to indulge in sweets, remind yourself of something positive about not doing so. Discipline is how you subject the urge to your willpower.

Say your affirmations under your breath; for example, "I want to enjoy my longevity in good health. I feel satisfied. It's just calories!" Use visualization to see yourself looking fit. These mind games will help boost your motivation to do the right thing. Those are the kinds of tricks that

Lucky Harry used to great effect. That is how you constantly saturate your mind with your main goal, and that process is called *autosuggestion*. You are constantly telling your mind what your goal is, and that is how it helps you to get it. The brain is very visual! It acts on what you present or will it to. It even does better if you emotionalize the goal—that is, present it with excitement. Passion will crystallize the goal into your heart. You'll see the activity as a passion rather than a chore. Why? Because when you develop passion for a goal, it's more self-motivating and empowering. At that point you actually feel good, even when you just think about doing it, let alone actually doing it.

Here is an example of a general and relatively clear goal: to have a Body Mass Index (BMI) of less than twenty-five. Ideally that is where your BMI should be. Let's say you want to lose ten pounds within a certain period of time. These two goals are specific enough that your brain can make sense out of them and take the daily action steps that move you forward to achieve success. These small steps have to be assimilated into your lifestyle in order to be effective.

Remember, a seven-pound weight loss will significantly drop your risk for the common killer diseases mentioned throughout this chapter.

Tip #3: What is Your Ideal Weight?

Your ideal weight is your healthy weight. Only about half of North Americans have a healthy weight. The other half has problems managing weight.

A healthy weight is different for everyone, and it depends on individual shape and height. We all lose and gain weight continuously. The key is to stick to a range that is healthy for you. In order to figure out the right range for you, you can look at the ratio of your weight to your height. This is call your Body Mass Index (BMI).

To discover your BMI, use the chart below. Locate the point where your height and weight intersect; that number is your BMI.

BMI Chart by BodyMassIndexChart.org

Weight [pounds]

Height [feet and inches]	100	110	120	130	140	150	160	170	180	190	200	210	220	230	240	250	260
4'6"	24	27	29	31	34	36	39	41	43	46	48	51	53	55	58	60	63
4'8"	22	25	27	29	31	34	36	38	40	43	45	47	49	52	54	56	58
4'10"	21	23	25	27	29	31	33	36	38	40	42	44	46	48	50	52	54
5'0"	20	21	23	25	27	29	31	33	35	37	39	41	43	45	47	49	51
5'2"	18	20	22	24	26	27	29	31	33	35	37	38	40	42	44	46	48
5'4"	17	19	21	22	24	26	27	29	31	33	34	36	38	39	41	43	45
5'6"	16	18	19	21	23	24	26	27	29	31	32	34	36	37	39	40	42
5'8"	15	17	18	20	21	23	24	26	27	29	30	32	33	35	36	38	40
5'10"	14	16	17	19	20	22	23	24	26	27	29	30	32	33	34	36	37
6'0"	14	15	16	18	19	20	22	23	24	26	27	28	30	31	33	34	35
6'2"	13	14	15	17	18	19	21	22	23	24	26	27	28	30	31	32	33
6'4"	12	13	15	16	17	18	19	21	22	23	24	26	27	28	29	30	32
6'6"	12	13	14	15	16	17	18	20	21	22	23	24	25	27	28	29	30
6'8"	11	12	13	14	15	16	18	19	20	21	22	23	24	25	26	27	29
6'10"	10	12	13	14	15	16	17	18	19	20	21	22	23	24	25	26	27
7'0"	10	11	12	13	14	15	16	17	18	19	20	21	22	23	24	25	26

Underweight   Normal Range   Overweight   Obese

(Source: www.bodymassindexchart.org)

To understand what your BMI means, look at how the chart below correlates with your level of risk for developing health problems.

Classification	BMI (kg/m^2)	Risk of developing health problems
Underweight	< 18.5	Increased
Normal Weight	18.5-24.9	Least
Overweight	25.0-29.9	Increased
Obese class I	30.0-34.9	High
Obese class II	35.0-39.9	Very High
Obese class III	> 40.0	Extremely High

Tip #4: Trick the Satiety Center

The satiety center for controlling appetite is in the brain. You can review its role on regulating the satisfaction and hunger mechanism discussed earlier in this chapter. There are many ways to trick it to seem like you are satisfied, so that the center will curb your appetite.

Remember that leptin and ghrelin hormones regulate your appetite. They sense the presence of food in the stomach, especially from the left side, where a lot of the nerves are found. So one way to mimic food in the stomach is to start your meal with a glass of water. That immediately begins to send the message to the satiety center of your brain that you are satisfied.

I had a big fight with Lucky Harry about this. He insisted on using a glass of juice to fill himself up instead. Well, it is a no-brainer that any substance will work, but the main reason for sticking to water is because it has no calories.

Also, chewing food thoroughly and slowly provides enough time to reach the left side of the stomach. That sends the message to the satiety center that you are satisfied.

Tip #5: What You Eat

This is another situation where you can play with your physiology. Your food choices are very important. How you combine carbohydrates and proteins help you lose weight and is a very important lever for moving your weight down. When your weight loss plan hits the wall, ask yourself whether you are eating the right foods in the right proportions.

During each meal, the key is to strive for a balance between the quantity of carbohydrates and proteins. Simply put food on your plate in a 1:1ratio, carbohydrates to proteins, because carbohydrates make your body secrete insulin, store fat, and make you crave more sugar, increasing your appetite. The craving and increase in appetite that comes after consuming sugars makes you eat more food rather than limit calorie intake, which should be the goal. Proteins, on the other hand, decrease your appetite. How? They make your body secrete glycagons, which modulate the effects of insulin and make your body burn more fat too. Note that vegetables and fruits are considered carbohydrates.

Tip #6: Think of Food as Medicine

We use medication when necessary, not for comfort. The food that we eat affects the hypothalamus, the command center in the brain, and our physiology, as in the cortisol mechanism. So avoid any unwanted calories from comfort food. Delete the empty calories from sweets, cakes, ice cream, etc.

This begins when you buy your food. You must buy only health foods!

Another important tip is to make it a habit to stop eating when you feel satisfied, not full. Light eating makes you feel light and energetic. When you eat a large meal, your body sends most of the blood to your stomach to digest the food. That leaves much less blood for your brain. Consequently, its oxygen level—the ultimate fuel of the body—falls too.

Tip #7: Eat Homemade Food

Our busy lifestyles have made many people turn to fast foods. Honestly, that has been one of the reasons for the obesity epidemic. It is an easy way out, but we pay with our thick waistlines. Processed foods have preservatives in them; salt is the main one. Salt makes our body retain water, which contributes to a host of ailments, including hypertension and weight gain. So when we make our own food, we can minimize the quantity of salt in it, as well as minimize the fat.

Tip #8: Daily Exercise

View exercise as medicine. It not only prevents but is also used as treatment for the common killer diseases discussed earlier. The benefits of making an hour of daily exercise part of your life are astronomical. But more importantly, exercise is a very important component of your weight-loss plan. Indeed, it is fair to say that you'll hardly succeed in keeping your weight under control without it. It is the key element on the expenditure aspect of energy.

My experience has been that controlling the amount of calories is the primary thing to do. Why? Because common sense tells me that it is easier to eat the modest amount of 1,500 calories a day and to exercise modestly to expend it, rather than eat a 2,500 calorie diet and then work so hard to exercise and lose it. Our sedentary lifestyles make exercising to burn calories necessary. After cutting down on the calories, exercise is the second important element in your arsenal for success.

Tip #9: Weight Lifting

If you want to loose weight, try lifting weights. One of the myths about losing weight is that weight lifting makes you bulkier. Well, there is some truth to it, because you can actually pick up some pounds with rigorous muscle building. But in the long run, you win because fat is burned in the muscle.

Tip #10: Supplements

There are lots of myths about supplements. Some people think that they make them lose weight. Generally they do not. A lot of them sound too good to be true. Some of them have sound scientific underpinnings to them, like the use of leptin products to lose weight, but as I explained earlier in this chapter, body functions are very complex. Having knowledge of one factor often is just the tip of the iceberg.

Sometimes the side effects are more than carrying the weight. Some people take them for the wrong reasons, but there are some good reasons to take them.

I know that a good number of people eat invariably poorly for all kinds of reasons, and because of our quest to look fit, some people do not consume adequate amounts of food. Many of the supplements that I recommend are rich in antioxidants, which help the body repair epithelial cell damage and protect us mainly against strokes , heart disease, and cancers. Some of them, like the B vitamins (in multivitamins) have lots of micro-nutrients like zinc and magnesium that are very important because they feed into many biochemical pathways.

Even some experts still hold the opinion that we get enough of these micro-nutrients from the food that we eat. I learned the same thing about fifteen years ago in medical school, but the tide has shifted in that respect on account of reputable evidence from studies.

The common over-the-counter nutritional supplements that people should be taking include multivitamins, omega 3, coenzyme Q10, and a fiber supplement. These are the basics; depending on your needs, you can take others. The amounts of vitamins in the multivitamins are for optimal functioning of the body. For example, there is a modest quantity of vitamin B-12, vitamin D, and calcium. But if you have deficiency in these nutrients, no problem; you can take some more vitamin D and calcium. A good example here is someone with osteoporosis. I greatly value the lives of the people that I help heal and will not do or say anything to jeopardize their well-being.

If your situation is a little complex to figure out, speak to a health care professional for help.

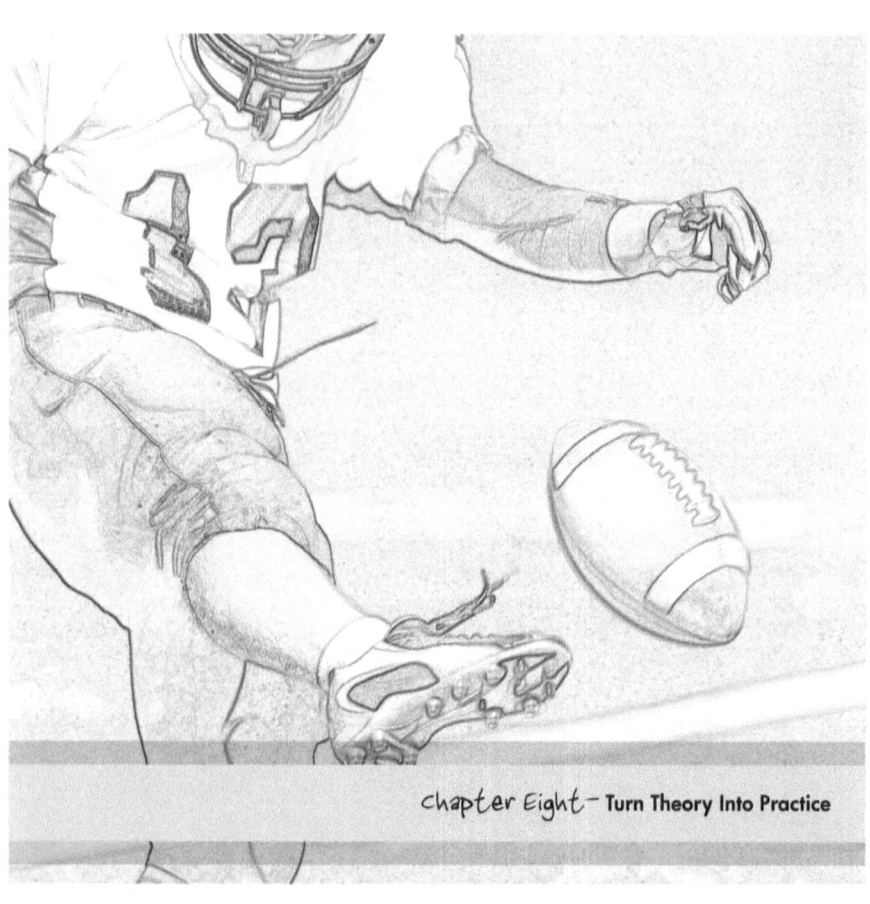

chapter Eight – **Turn Theory Into Practice**

Chapter Eight

Turn Theory Into Practice

Command Your Destiny

When Lucky Harry came to see me, he was totally discouraged about his life. It was his wife who wanted him to see the doctor. And he had to, because he needed cardiac rehabilitation in order to get back into shape. Not only that, he needed my release in order for his employer to allow him back to work after the heart attack.

At least in Lucky Harry's mind, he thought that he was a failure because the family tree was to blame for his triple whammy of diabetes, obesity, and heart disease. He felt so powerless because he thought that he was too fat to exercise, and he held many other self-defeating ideas. He was marching himself down the same negative path as his father, which lead to the heart attack that took his life.

But I kept reminding Lucky Harry that he was really lucky; his life was spared despite the massive heart attack he had. And rather than wallow in self-pity, he should seize the bull by the horns and defy the family tree.

Lucky Harry loved building an emotional cell for himself. He saw himself as a victim of the family tree. He definitely programmed his mind to fail. I knew that the key to turning the situation around was to help him overcome the negative conditioning that he had built throughout his life. Until he changed the self-limiting beliefs that he had, he could not move forward. It took many months of inspiring him on how to turn theory into practice.

Well, some people are like Lucky Harry. They are very well informed about what to do in order to be in good shape. The trouble is that they do not do it. That is why we have a very large gap between knowledge and action.

But how do we get what we want? This may sound simple, but it's profound to say that we start by telling ourselves what we want. That is the willing process. That is how we identify with what we want. It is through that conscious or unconscious process that we shape our thoughts, behaviors, and actions over time to eventually get what we want. Does it always work? No. But that is the process. It involves the creation of new habits and letting go of the ones that we do not want.

When it comes to proper conditioning, the subconscious mind is responsible. But it depends on the conscious mind for making the right choices about what to do. The subconscious function of the mind simply executes what the conscious mind impresses on it. So for optimal functioning, they both have to be synchronized.

The myths and false beliefs that Lucky Harry had were hampering his efforts.

Take, for example, his belief that he was too fat to exercise. That belief is a function of the conscious, reasoning mind. And that confuses the subconscious mind, rather than reinforcing it. In order to strengthen its ability to execute, the subconscious mind should be told what to do in an unwavering manner.

You can appreciate why clear goals are crucial. People like Lucky Harry are often vague in terms of what they want. The mixed messages impressed on the subconscious mind makes it dither! Winners think clearly, with confidence and boldness, about what they want. Consequently, their goals are also clear. They are never vague—unless intentionally!

So, demystifying false beliefs and making clear the benefits of healthy living to Lucky Harry was important. Awareness of what is right dispels some of the false beliefs. Also, knowing the benefits of healthy living helps strengthen our resolve for acting.

It was both very challenging and humbling for Lucky Harry to know that he was among the half of North Americans who are having trouble controlling their weight. In some ways, it was reassuring to him that he was not alone. But it put pressure on him to try to move himself to the positive half of that scale with the people who are succeeding in managing their weight.

I highlighted that because about half of his obesity was environmentally determined, he could change that part. Evidence suggests that the causes of obesity are at least 50 percent genetic. So he does in fact own part of the blame, along with his family tree.

I had no problem confronting Lucky Harry about his obesity. As a health care professional, I have observed that this problem is often ignored because of the social stigma associated with discussing it. Obesity is among the most important public health problems in North America, if not the most important. Not only is it an epidemic, but it more than doubles our risk for heart disease, which is a major killer.

Obesity is defined as a person having a Body Mass Index (BMI) of more than 30 kg/m² or 20 percent higher than their ideal body weight. The prevalence of obesity in North America is about 23 percent in adults. When combined with those who are overweight (a BMI of 25 to 29.9) that percentage jumps to a staggering 50 percent of adults who are carrying excess weight.

Note that children are of particular concern because their obesity rates are on the rise. About 25 percent of children are overweight. Also, the rate of type II diabetes in children has increased significantly in the last decade.[24]

What is the solution? The solution is to turn the theory that we already know into practice. Having a lifestyle plan is the key to healthy living. Becoming a model of restraint regarding what we consume plus regular daily exercise are the critical elements in our arsenal for success and healthy living.

Why? Because modern living often results in a sedentary lifestyle. This is compounded by the fact that most of our day jobs involve little or no physical activity. Physical inactivity can cause early death through the weakening of our major organs, like the heart, causing chronic disease that eventually kills.

On the other hand, regular exercise improves both our health and well-being. It improves our mood, makes our heart stronger, and reduces stress-related diseases. It also builds our energy and maintains our ideal body weight. It is our main way of burning calories in order to maintain a fair balance between calories in and out. In an affluent society, our problem

---

24   Tallia, Alfred F., Dennis A. Cardone, David F. Howarth. *Swanson's Family Practice Review*. C.V. Mosby. 2000.

is trying to resist the urge to over-consume calories. These are the reasons why our action steps for healthy living are directed toward turning the theory that we already know to a practice.

Action Steps

Action Step #1: Think Smart

My concept of thinking smart requires using your brain as an ally for succeeding. Why? Because our brain acts on what it sees! That is how we get what we get. So we have to first will what we want by making the request to our subconscious mind through our reasoning mind. Our conscious mind makes decisions that are impressed onto the subconscious, which holds them as memory or belief and then executes them in turn.

So you have to ask or tell your subconscious mind what to do. You have to assume the role of what you want. You have to see yourself with the happy ending. That is how you induce your subconscious mind to act on your behalf. You can do it voluntarily or involuntarily. The basis of the process is the use of your imagination and your thoughts. That is why thinking and imagination are so important. They initiate as well as move you toward what you desire. How? These processes help you identify with what you want—playing the role.

The word *autosuggestion* could be used to describe what I am talking about. It means telling yourself something specific, voluntarily or involuntarily. It determines your internal dialogue, whether it's positive or negative. These are the two main filters that people use. They either have a negative or positive thought pattern, determined by what they tell themselves, which establishes their perception and how they interpret the world around them.

The key to identifying with what you want is acknowledging that your thoughts, behaviors, actions, and feelings flow from your internal dialogue. Again, this could be either voluntary or involuntary; when someone's predominant filter is set on the negative, their pattern of thought follows it. They are likely to remember the dark side, including bad memories of the past, as opposed to remembering the bright side. No wonder such thoughts tend to push people into an emotional hole! Quite often people feel sad because they think thoughts of inadequacy or feel despair for a real or perceived failure.

When I first met Lucky Harry, he was not able to answer simple questions, like how many times he exercised each week and how many calories he consumed each day. He was not actively playing the role to become what he wanted! He was very vague about what he wanted. He was not specific. And as a result, so were the requests that he impressed onto his subconscious mind. So he conditioned himself to fail.

In order to stop him from going down the wrong path, I taught him how to manage the willing process to create specific and clear goals, turn them into affirmations, and impress his subconscious mind with them all through the day, especially just before falling asleep, because his subconscious is more receptive at that time, when much of the noise of the reasoning mind is turned off.

The best way to find out how many calories you need each day is to match how much you eat to your ideal weight. Why? Because it depends on how active you are and whether your job is physical or not. But having knowledge of what the average person eats is important too. The average person needs about 2,500 calories a day. To lose weight, you can reduce the amount of food that you eat down about 1,500 calories.

One of the mistakes that some people make is to drastically reduce their calories, known as crash dieting, to around the range of 500 calories per day. That is very bad, because it sends your body into shock, releasing cortisol, the stress hormone, shutting down your metabolism. So, rather than losing weight, you hit a snag. This is not good for the body because it does not help you maintain your ideal weight. But even worse, long-term stress causes the pituitary gland in the brain to stimulate the adrenal gland to release adrenaline and cortisol. They feed the vicious cycle of making you feel more stress, as well as increasing your chances of developing stress-related diseases like high blood pressure, high cholesterol, diabetes, obesity, strokes, and heart attack—all of which are major killers.

Lucky Harry made affirmations that he repeated all day long to himself about what he wanted. He would say, "I exercise everyday. I exercise one hour each day. I get out of bed at 6:00 a.m. each day." This is how he changed the things that he was telling himself every day. That is how he overcame the negative or limiting beliefs that were holding him back.

I am sure that there are other people like Lucky Harry with distorted beliefs that govern their lives. When we mentally accept these limiting beliefs, our subconscious mind acts accordingly. This is why belief is so powerful. As soon as we entertain an idea mentally, the subconscious mind acts accordingly. In order to reverse negative trends, we have to first change the way we think. Our actions, behaviors, and feelings will follow! If our lifestyle plan is what we want, then we keep on reinforcing it. If its not what we want, then our power lies in changing that lifestyle, beginning with our thoughts.

Action Step #2: Choose Good Habits

Lucky Harry now understands the significance of clear and specific goals. He used to joke with me that it is better late than never; even though he learned this in his sixties, it will still be of great value in his quest for healthy living. His example can carry on to his children and grandchildren, creating a healthy new heredity.

He learned that setting clear and specific goals meant telling the brain what he wanted in life; otherwise, how would it know? He told me that he had never thought of it that way. But it made sense to him. The simple act of figuring out your goal helps the prefrontal area of the brain to sustain attention; otherwise it is wasted. Your actions become scattered, not focused. Imagine trying to shoot at a flock of ducks flying in the air with your eyes closed!

He learned that your whole life avails to nothing when your reasoning mind and the subconscious mind are not in harmony. That is why the habit of aligning your thoughts with your goals is important. He realized that such conditioning is important in orchestrating the behaviors and actions that lead to success.

Lucky Harry realized that he had been his own worst enemy. He was an obstacle to living the lifestyle that will lead to long-term health. He let go of the assumption that he was too fat to exercise!

He had fallen into the trap that a good number of people do. Harry tried crash dieting, reducing his caloric intake to 500 calories per day. It drove Lucky Harry crazy. I explained to him how he was shutting down his metabolism and preventing the body from breaking down the food that he was eating.

In creating the habit of healthy living, a lifestyle plan or change is needed for long-term success. The short-term action of resisting the urge to over-consume only works when extended for a long period.

My small bang theory emphasizes the power of small steps and their compounding effect over time. It is very powerful to compare short-term pleasure from the cakes or sweets to the long-term benefit of a healthy life, hopefully leading to avoiding those calories to ward off being overweight or developing diabetes from the stress that too many sweets place on your pancreas, which eventually burns out that organ. Since sugars stimulate the pancreas to produce insulin, large loads of sugars create undue pressure on it. Eventually, as burnout occurs, it is not able produce as much insulin as it used to. Sugars that are not being broken down accumulate due to lack of insulin. That describes diabetes.

So what Lucky Harry did was fill his mind with positive thoughts and images of what he wanted. His wish was to look fit, so he implanted that image in his mind. He felt good when he passed on dessert. He told himself that dessert was just calories that he did not need. He also visualized himself at the finish line when he exercised for one hour each day. He also brought his wife into the picture because she was a major source of his support.

So Lucky Harry had his new script for life: the new habits that he wanted to make happen. That was the first step. He made them into simple affirmations that he could repeat under his breath all day long and shortly before falling asleep at night.

He learned that the key to making the right move and establishing the right habits was to make the conscious mind and subconscious mind cooperate. So he stopped fighting himself. When he went to bed before, he used to blame his medical problems on his family tree. He was coiled like a spring, and angry, and that disrupted his sleep, making him even more frustrated. Now he knew that all he needed to do was crowd out the old habits by simply repeating the new script to himself all day long. That was the best way to break the old habit, not fighting with it! Constant practice over time will shape thoughts, behaviors, and actions.

At first, this sort of conditioning is done consciously. That is why the reasoning mind is principally involved. But with time, the subconscious mind reacts to the ideas that challenge it, so it executes the action. After some time, the particular habit becomes automatic, or second nature.

As you can see, the basis of this process is use of imagination. We can use this technique to foster or change any habit we want to change. Creating a blueprint for the new habit and saturating our mind with it simply crowds out and replaces the undesired one.

Action Step #3: Pull the Trigger

I met with Lucky Harry and his wife only after his wife forced him to come and see me. He had already assumed that he was a failure. There are other people out there like him. He definitely had already conditioned himself to fail. I spoke to both of them. I realized that he had the destructive habit of procrastination. He wouldn't have come to the doctor had it not been because of the scare he got from having a heart attack. And his encouraging wife may also have had something to do with it!

It irked me that someone in his sixties was still such a low performer. He did not understand some of the basic rules for success. Many months of my coaching and the use of positive affirmations transformed him into a high performer. He became decisive. Pulling the trigger means that you should willfully begin an action. All the knowledge in the world would not take him anywhere if Lucky Harry did not learn to pull the trigger!

I discovered that the most limiting factor keeping him from achieving success in the area of healthy living was the false beliefs that he entertained. That was how he conditioned himself to fail. This was the turning point for Lucky Harry. He realized that those limiting beliefs had to be changed if he was to build a healthy lifestyle. What we think we create. It is the most powerful force that humans possess. Our thoughts dwell on what we believe in, and over time our subconscious mind reacts to our reasoning mind and brings our goal to pass.

Mentally, he saw himself in that imaginary role. He thought of the happy ending. He infused himself with excitement. How? He drew a composite picture of himself showing how he wanted to look. It was a thin, smiling figure with the long strides of a marathoner. This is how Lucky Harry emotionalized exercise and other behaviors and actions that helped him move forward to achieve his long-term goal.

All through the day and shortly before falling asleep, he said to himself that he was very confident that he could be amongst the half of the population that had a handle on their weight. Indeed, he fired himself up more by acting as if he had already succeeded. That reinforced the subconscious mind to deliver the results.

Motivation is the force that moves us to action. It is an emotional state. Most of it comes from within. Lucky Harry's wife was a very strong external source of motivation. But the crux of the matter is that without the individual summoning up the forces from within, nothing will happen.

Lucky Harry's wife preached over many years to deaf ears. He did not act accordingly until the wake-up call from a heart attack. He was obliged to pay attention because he needed cardiac rehabilitation to go back to work.

Exercise is medicine in that respect, because it increases the survival rate of heart attack victims by 50 percent. That is huge! It also reduces the risk of the other major killer diseases that we have discussed throughout the book. Daily exercise is used as a treatment for those common diseases:

heart attack, stroke, hypertension, anxiety, stress, depression, and many others.

Motivation is a strong urge or tendency toward or away from a goal or object. High performers have a very high creative power. They do not wait for external incentives in order to perform. They can also resist the negative urges that could distract them from their goal. And fear can either stimulate or serve as an inhibitor to achieving a goal. Despite the scare from a heart attack, Lucky Harry could have chosen to refrain from action, had his wife not encouraged him.

There are more than a few reasons for seeing a doctor before starting an exercise regimen. If you are not sure about your level of fitness, then see a health care professional. Sometimes tests may discover medical problems that could be related with your being overweight.

Pulling the trigger is a very effective way to overcome procrastination. It is also a way to push yourself out of your comfort zone. A pattern of positive achievement will help you develop even more passion toward your goal.

Action Step #4: Go the Extra Mile

Lucky Harry has been transformed from a low to a high performer. One very important distinction between low and high performers is that the latter are very hardworking. They are not lazy. Going the extra mile means doing a little more than the average person. It has many advantages. One of them is that it sharpens your competitive edge, and it makes you stand out in the crowd.

Lucky Harry told me that he walked an extra mile even when he felt that his strength was gone. He said that there were days when he felt like quitting the treadmill halfway, but he resisted the urge. He filled his mind with the positive picture that he drew of himself smiling and taking big strides. Looking fit in that picture fired him up. One of the pictures was hanging on the wall in the basement where he worked out on the treadmill. He also hung one of them around his neck when he went for his walks. He told people that he used to look like that and was very determined to get back to the way he was in his thirties.

His wife used to say that it was a little too ambitious for a guy in his sixties to want to look thirty again. But I told her that a little bit of ambition would not hurt the man, but it would help fire him up! Simple as it seemed, lack of any ambition for something better was why he had been stuck with obesity for such a long time. So once he started being imaginative, why not let him liberate himself from the self-made prison and move forward—attaining freedom, well-being, and healthy living and leaving his comfort zone, which had provided a false sense of comfort. Once he gained a measure of confidence, he could then sit and laugh at himself a little and at least talk about the past with humor.

He used to ask me why ice cream tasted better at midnight. I thought it was a weird question, because I did not know why he would be having ice cream at that time. But as I started to get to know him better, I discovered that he tiptoed to the freezer in the middle of the night when his wife was sleeping. The light bulb in my head came on as I connected the dots. The obvious explanation was that the stress that he was feeling because he was worrying about his wife suddenly waking up and catching him with a bowl of ice cream in the middle of the night initiated the cortisol mechanism. This mechanism eventually lead to a heightened appetite and food cravings, which Lucky Harry interpreted as the ice cream tasting better.

Since he could not resist the urge to indulge in midnight ice cream, his wife could have helped Lucky Harry indirectly rather than laying down the rule for him not to have it. She could have just stopped buying it for his sake. Finally she did just that.

The move toward making healthy food choices starts at the supermarket. We have to carefully choose what we buy and bring home. Why buy stuff that we know that is not fit for consumption? We just torture ourselves! Just making the decision to buy what is right is half the battle. Most of the people I speak to know what to buy and eat—they just don't do it.

Goals are the fire-starters in our lives. They actually help pace and program our lives when we make the commitment to act. A goal is a pledge that must be backed by discipline and hard work in order to be realized. The only true test of discipline is action. So we have to consistently act in order to achieve results.

I have already discussed the small bang theory in detail. It means that the seemingly small steps we take everyday are eventually compounded, and that is how success comes about. Quite often procrastinators underestimate the power of small steps, and they want to get it all done at once. But it never happens. It is like wanting to leave your house for a destination, but you wait for all the lights to turn green before you start your journey. Lucky Harry was like that!

Each time you decline dessert, you are saving yourself some calories; over years that becomes a lot. Be imaginative. Try to visualize a mountain of dessert that you decline during one year, and see how many thousands of calories you spare yourself!

Also, ten minutes of exercise a day is better than none at all. You do not have to do one hour in one go. No. You can do ten minutes several times a day. That is what Lucky Harry assimilated into his lifestyle.

Choose any exercise that you find fun. Make the move right now! Action steps overcome procrastination. And once started, the momentum begins to build.

Measure your progress. It helps you improve your score. It raises your awareness of how much more you can do in order to reduce the gap between knowledge and action for the same reason that we count calories. It raises your awareness about the number of calories that you are eating each day. And awareness is a key step in either reinforcing your lifestyle plan or changing it, if need be.

Lucky Harry's success came because he became imaginative and decided to choose good habits that helped him achieve healthy living. His cooperation was necessary. He turned the corner and achieved excellent health—something he always thought of as just a dream.

We all can do what he did if we follow the simple action steps I have laid out in this chapter. But recognize the fact that in the end, the onus is on you to act. No one can do it for you. In order to succeed, you have to become an instrument of positive influence; otherwise, it will not work. Your intentions have to be followed by actions in order to achieve results.

It is possible to sing the same song, yet dance differently. That is why your real measure is your actions, not your words. True commitment comes from the heart; the passion that you carry dissolves the apparent obstacles that hold you back. But in order to deliver results, you must consistently match your thoughts with appropriate actions. That is how you control your destiny. Sometimes it takes a long time to find your strength zone. Once you enter your strength zone, stay there!

About the Author

Dr. Alfred Nkut, M.D., is an accomplished physician, entrepreneur, and philanthropist, with an avid interest in leadership. His experiences studying medicine in Cameroon and in his family medical residency in Canada have shown him that self-improvement, especially development of character goals, is not emphasized in most formal educational systems. For this reason, he became increasingly interested in studying, learning, growing, and researching to provide additional insight into the subject of leadership.

Dr. Nkut sees every day as an opportunity to add value, not only to his own life but to the lives of others as well. He has founded the Skylimit Corporation to make a difference in people's lives and the Equity Trust Finance in Cameroon, West Africa, with the goal of poverty relief.

The more he learns about and understands the areas of leadership and success, the more passion he has for sharing that knowledge and for encouraging those who wish to improve their lives. He knows of no better way to get a kick out of life than to give, because for him giving is receiving; it is love—and that's how you make your way to "heaven."

Dr. Nkut and his wife, Dr. Elaine Blacklock, both practice medicine in Greater Sudbury, Ontario, Canada, and along with their children, Jacob and Ruthie, are proud to call the city home.

www.alfrednkut.com